T0130822

# Minimally Invasive Gynecologic Surgery

*Editors*

TED LEE
NICOLE DONNELLAN

# OBSTETRICS AND GYNECOLOGY CLINICS OF NORTH AMERICA

www.obgyn.theclinics.com

*Consulting Editor*
WILLIAM F. RAYBURN

June 2022 • Volume 49 • Number 2

**ELSEVIER**

1600 John F. Kennedy Boulevard • Suite 1800 • Philadelphia, Pennsylvania, 19103-2899

http://www.theclinics.com

**OBSTETRICS AND GYNECOLOGY CLINICS OF NORTH AMERICA Volume 49 Number 2
June 2022 ISSN 0889-8545, ISBN-13: 978-0-323-98745-5**

Editor: Kerry Holland
Developmental Editor: Hannah Almira Lopez

*Obstetrics and Gynecology Clinics* (ISSN 0889-8545) is published quarterly by Elsevier Inc., 360 Park Avenue South, New York, NY 10010-1710. Months of issue are March, June, September, and December. Periodicals postage paid at New York, NY, and additional mailing offices. Subscription price per year is $345.00 (US individuals), $963.00 (US institutions), $100.00 (US students), $416.00 (Canadian individuals), $982.00 (Canadian institutions), $100.00 (Canadian students), $473.00 (international individuals), $982.00 (international institutions), and $225.00 (international students). To receive student/resident rate, orders must be accompanied by name of affiliated institution, date of term, and the signature of program/residency coordinator on institution letterhead. Orders will be billed at individual rate until proof of status is received. Foreign air speed delivery is included in all *Clinics* subscription prices. All prices are subject to change without notice. POSTMASTER: Send address changes to *Obstetrics and Gynecology Clinics*, Elsevier Health Sciences Division, Subscription Customer Service, 3251 Riverport Lane, Maryland Heights, MO 63043. **Customer Service: Telephone: 1-800-654-2452 (U.S. and Canada); 314-447-8871 (outside U.S. and Canada). Fax: 314-447-8029. E-mail: journalscustomerservice-usa@elsevier.com (for print support); journalsonlinesupport-usa@elsevier. com (for online support).**

*Reprints.* For copies of 100 or more of articles in this publication, please contact the Commercial Reprints Department, Elsevier Inc., 360 Park Avenue South, New York, New York 10010-1710. Tel.: 212-633-3874; Fax: 212-633-3820; E-mail: reprints@elsevier.com.

*Obstetrics and Gynecology Clinics of North America* is also published in Spanish by McGraw-Hill Interamericana Editores S.A., P.O. Box 5-237, 06500, Mexico; in Portuguese by Reichmann and Affonso Editores, Rio de Janeiro, Brazil; and in Greek by Paschalidis Medical Publications, Athens, Greece.

*Obstetrics and Gynecology Clinics of North America is covered in MEDLINE/PubMed (Index Medicus), Excerpta Medica, Current Concepts/Clinical Medicine, Science Citation Index, BIOSIS, CINAHL, and ISI/BIOMED.*

# Contributors

## CONSULTING EDITOR

**WILLIAM F. RAYBURN, MD, MBA**
Affiliate Professor, Department of Obstetrics and Gynecology and College of Graduate Studies Medical University of South Carolina Charleston, South Carolina Emeritus Distinguished Professor, Department of Obstetrics and Gynecology University of New Mexico School of Medicine Albuquerque, New Mexico

## EDITORS

**TED LEE, MD**
Director, Minimally Invasive Gynecologic Surgery, Clinical Professor, Department of Obstetrics, Gynecology, and Reproductive Sciences, University of Pittsburgh School of Medicine, UPMC Magee-Womens Hospital, Pittsburgh, Pennsylvania, USA

**NICOLE DONNELLAN, MD**
Associate Professor, Associate PD, Obstetrics, Gynecology, and Reproductive Sciences Residency, Associate PD, FMIGS, Department of Obstetrics, Gynecology, and Reproductive Sciences, University of Pittsburgh School of Medicine, UPMC Magee-Womens Hospital, Pittsburgh, Pennsylvania, USA

## AUTHORS

**SAWSAN AS-SANIE, MD, MPH**
Department of Obstetrics and Gynecology, University of Michigan, Ann Arbor, Michigan, USA

**PATRICIA GIGLIO AYERS, MD**
Resident Physician, Department of Obstetrics and Gynecology, The Warren Alpert Medical School of Brown University, Women & Infants Hospital, Providence, Rhode Island, USA

**BRIANA L. BAXTER, MD**
Fellow, Minimally Invasive Gynecologic Surgery, Division of Gynecologic Specialty Surgery, Department of Obstetrics and Gynecology, Columbia University Irving Medical Center, New York, New York, USA

**JUBILEE BROWN, MD**
Division of Gynecologic Oncology, Levine Cancer Institute at Atrium Health, Charlotte, North Carolina, USA

**LISA CHAO, MD**
Assistant Professor of Obstetrics and Gynecology, Associate Director of Fellowship in MIGS, Division of Gynecology, Department of Obstetrics and Gynecology, The University of Texas Southwestern Medical Center, Dallas, Texas, USA

**RICHARD COCKRUM, MD**
Clinical Instructor, Department of Obstetrics and Gynecology, NorthShore University
HealthSystem, Evanston, Illinois, USA; Department of Obstetrics and Gynecology,
University of Chicago, Pritzker School of Medicine, Chicago, Illinois, USA

**JON IVAR EINARSSON, MD, PhD, MPH**
Chief, Division of Minimally Invasive Gynecology, Professor, Harvard Medical School,
Boston, Massachusetts, USA

**CHRISTINE E. FOLEY, MD**
Assistant Professor, Department of Obstetrics and Gynecology, The Warren Alpert
Medical School of Brown University, Women & Infants Hospital, Providence, Rhode
Island, USA

**JENNA GALE MD, MSC, FRCSC**
Assistant Professor, University of Ottawa, Clinical Investigator, Ottawa Hospital Research
Institute, Physician, Department of Obstetrics, Gynecology and Newborn Care, The
Ottawa Hospital, Associate Physician, Ottawa Fertility Centre, Ottawa, Ontario, Canada

**RICHARD S. GUIDO, MD**
Professor of Obstetrics and Gynecology, Kanbour Chair in Gynecology, Department of
Obstetrics, Gynecology and Reproductive Sciences, UPMC Magee-Womens Hospital,
Pittsburgh, Pennsylvania, USA

**SHABNAM GUPTA, MD**
Clinical Fellow in Minimally Invasive Gynecologic Surgery, Brigham & Women's Hospital,
Harvard Medical School, Boston, Massachusetts, USA

**HYE-CHUN HUR, MD, MPH**
Division of Gynecologic Specialty Surgery, Associate Professor, Department of
Obstetrics and Gynecology, Columbia University Irving Medical Center, New York, New
York, USA

**KIMBERLY KHO, MD, MPH**
Associate Professor of Obstetrics and Gynecology, Director of Fellowship in MIGS,
Division of Gynecology, Department of Obstetrics and Gynecology, The University of
Texas Southwestern Medical Center, Dallas, Texas, USA

**TED T. LEE, MD**
Director, Minimally Invasive Gynecologic Surgery, Clinical Professor, Department of
Obstetrics, Gynecology, and Reproductive Sciences, University of Pittsburgh School of
Medicine, UPMC Magee-Womens Hospital, Pittsburgh, Pennsylvania, USA

**BRITTANY LEES, MD**
Division of Gynecologic Oncology, Levine Cancer Institute at Atrium Health, Charlotte,
North Carolina, USA

**EMILY LIN, MD**
Fellow, Minimally Invasive Gynecologic Surgery, Division of Gynecology, Department of
Obstetrics and Gynecology, The University of Texas Southwestern Medical Center,
Dallas, Texas, USA

**NASH S. MOAWAD, MD, MS**
Associate Professor and Chief, Division of Minimally Invasive Gynecologic Surgery,
Department of Obstetrics and Gynecology, University of Florida College of Medicine,
Gainesville, Florida, USA

**REINA NAKAMURA, DO**
Department of Physical Medicine and Rehabilitation, University of Michigan, Ann Arbor, Michigan, USA

**HANNAH PALIN, MD**
Fellow, Minimally Invasive Gynecologic Surgery, Mayo Clinic, Jacksonville, Florida, USA

**JAMES K. ROBINSON III, MD, MS, FACOG**
Vice Chair, Women's and Infants' Services, Director, Minimally Invasive Gynecologic Surgery, Associate Director, AAGL Fellowship in Minimally Invasive Gynecologic Surgery, MedStar Washington Hospital Center, Washington, DC, USA

**ANDREW SCHREPF, PhD**
Department of Anesthesiology, University of Michigan, Ann Arbor, Michigan, USA

**SUKHBIR SONY SINGH MD, FRCSC, FACOG**
Professor, University of Ottawa, Director, AAGL Fellowship in Minimally Invasive Gynecologic Surgery, E. Jolly Research Chair in Gynecologic Surgery, Ottawa Hospital Research Institute, Chair of the Department of Obstetrics, Gynecology and Newborn Care, The Ottawa Hospital, Ottawa, Ontario, Canada

**LAUREN N. THOLEMEIER, MD**
Department of Obstetrics and Gynecology, Cedars-Sinai Medical Center, Los Angeles, California, USA

**SARA R. TILL, MD, MPH**
Department of Obstetrics and Gynecology, University of Michigan, Ann Arbor, Michigan, USA

**MIREILLE D. TRUONG, MD**
Department of Obstetrics and Gynecology, Cedars-Sinai Medical Center, Los Angeles, California, USA

**FRANK TU, MD, MPH**
Clinical Professor, Vice Chair of Quality, Division Director for Gynecology, Department of Obstetrics and Gynecology, NorthShore University HealthSystem, Evanston, Illinois, USA; Department of Obstetrics and Gynecology, University of Chicago, Pritzker School of Medicine, Chicago, Illinois, USA

**ANNA ZELIVIANSKAIA, MD**
Fellow in Minimally Invasive Gynecologic Surgery, Department of Obstetrics and Gynecology, MedStar Washington Hospital Center and Georgetown, University School of Medicine, Washington, DC, USA

# Contents

Foreword: Minimally Invasive Gynecologic Surgery: Improving Outcomes and
Recovery While Reducing Discomfort and Cost                                    xiii

William F. Rayburn

Preface: Holistic Approach to Minimally Invasive Gynecologic Surgery            xv

Ted Lee and Nicole Donnellan

Approach to Diagnosis and Management of Chronic Pelvic Pain in Women:
Incorporating Chronic Overlapping Pain Conditions in Assessment and Management   219

Sara R. Till, Reina Nakamura, Andrew Schrepf, and Sawsan As-Sanie

Chronic pelvic pain (CPP) is multifactorial in etiology and heterogeneous in presentation. Identification of all pain contributors is essential for successful management. Chronic overlapping pain conditions (COPCs) are a specified group of chronic pain conditions that commonly co-occur in patients. We briefly review individual COPCs and highlight risk factors and mechanisms that appear to be applicable across COPCs. We review evaluation and communication strategies that may help establish a productive therapeutic relationship between clinicians and patients. Management should include treatment of peripheral pain generators as well as co-occurring psychological conditions and central sensitization when present.

A Practical Approach to Fertility Considerations in Endometriosis Surgery         241

Jenna Gale and Sukhbir Sony Singh

Endometriosis surgery requires thoughtful consideration and planning for those with infertility or those who wish to conceive in the future. Clinical history, examination, imaging, and fertility assessment can help plan, prepare and provide goal-directed surgical interventions when required. Further understanding of the benefits and limitations of surgery on future fertility outcomes is essential for those who provide care for patients with endometriosis. Endometriosis is a prevalent gynecologic condition, especially among patients with infertility. Studies demonstrate that, from a fertility perspective, surgery for endometriosis likely has a beneficial impact on the chance of spontaneous conception; however, selecting the appropriate surgical candidate can be challenging. To make a fully informed decision with regard to surgery, it is important to determine the patient's fertility goals and to conduct a thorough workup. Among patients with endometriosis-related infertility, first-line-assisted reproductive technology (ART) is generally preferred over surgery. Specific consideration in cases of minimal or mild endometriosis, ovarian endometrioma(s), and deep endometriosis (DE) are required for targeted counseling. Patients with symptoms significantly impacting their quality of life (QOL), or indications to proceed with surgery (ie, risk of malignancy, organ obstruction, or dysfunction) are best managed with surgical care by an experienced team. Surgery should be considered cautiously given the risks of damage to ovarian reserve, adhesions, and surgical complications. Risk of damage to ovarian reserve is a particularly important consideration among patients with endometrioma(s), with or without low ovarian reserve, and surgical complications are especially prevalent among patients undergoing surgery for bowel endometriosis. Goal-directed surgical treatment, as opposed to the traditional perspective of complete disease eradication, may be of particular importance among selected patients whereby fertility is a priority.

### Hysterectomy for Chronic Pelvic Pain                                   257

Richard Cockrum and Frank Tu

For well selected patients with chronic pelvic pain (CPP), 74% to 95% of women will report complete or significant improvement in pain after hysterectomy. A thoughtful history, examination, and review of imaging can improve success by linking pain complaints to discrete pathology, menstrual activity, or uterine tenderness. All patients with CPP should be evaluated for chronic overlapping pain conditions (COPCs) (eg, irritable bowel syndrome (IBS), fibromyalgia) and risk factors for persistent pain or chronic postsurgical pain (eg, depression, pain catastrophizing, central sensitization), and offered treatment as indicated. There are special considerations for preoperative planning and enhanced recovery for patients with chronic pain.

### Role of Robotic Surgery in Benign Gynecology                          273

Mireille D. Truong and Lauren N. Tholemeier

Since Food and Drug Administration approval in 2005, use of the robotic device in gynecologic surgery has continued to increase. There has been a growing number of applications in various surgical specialties including gynecology, and the surgical robot has been established as an additional surgical tool for performing minimally invasive gynecologic surgery. In this article, the authors review the development of robotic gynecologic surgery, clinical considerations, and future directions.

### Laparoscopic Abdominal Cerclage                                       287

Shabnam Gupta and Jon Ivar Einarsson

Cervical insufficiency is a well-established cause of infant morbidity and mortality. Recommended treatment of cervical insufficiency includes a procedure in which a stitch, termed a cerclage, is placed around the cervix to keep it closed. Abdominal cerclage is the preferred approach for patients with refractory cervical insufficiency or anatomic limitations to vaginal cerclage placement. Laparoscopic abdominal cerclage has many benefits over an open approach and has been increasingly performed over the last 20 years due to surgeon skillset and improved neonatal survival compared with repeat vaginal cerclage. Laparoscopic abdominal cerclage is a highly effective, well-tolerated surgical treatment of selected patients.

**Emerging Treatment Options for Fibroids**     299

Briana L. Baxter, Hye-Chun Hur, and Richard S. Guido

Leiomyomas (fibroids) are common, usually benign, monoclonal tumors that arise from the uterine myometrium. Clinical presentation is variable; some patients are asymptomatic, whereas others experience heavy menstrual bleeding, pain, bulk symptoms, and/or alterations in fertility. Previously, treatment options for fibroids were largely surgical. However, over the last decade, options have grown to include many medical and procedural options that allow for uterine and fertility preservation. Clinicians must become familiar with these options to adequately counsel patients desiring treatment of fibroids.

**Office Hysteroscopy: Setting up Your Practice for Success**     315

Anna Zelivianskaia and James K. Robinson III

 Video content accompanies this article at http://www.obgyn. theclinics.com.

Office hysteroscopy is a highly effective procedure for the evaluation and treatment of intrauterine pathology. The "see and treat" approach allows for patient treatment with the fewest amount of patient visits. The development of smaller cameras and instruments, as well as the employment of a vaginoscopy technique, has led to greater tolerability of office hysteroscopy and significant success of the "see and treat" approach. Most office hysteroscopic procedures can be accomplished with minimal premedication. There are many choices for equipment types and sterilization methods for the office hysteroscopy practice. Reimbursement for office hysteroscopy has improved, but economic challenges remain.

**Hysteroscopic Myomectomy**     329

Nash S. Moawad and Hannah Palin

 Video content accompanies this article at http://www.obgyn. theclinics.com.

Hysteroscopic myomectomy is the treatment of choice for symptomatic submucosal myomas, with excellent success rate and low complication rate.

**Evaluation and Management of Common Intraoperative and Postoperative Complications in Gynecologic Endoscopy**     355

Brittany Lees and Jubilee Brown

Gynecologic laparoscopy is a safe and effective route of surgery for many types of procedures. The potential for injury does exist, and prevention and timely recognition of complications are essential for maintaining the quality and safety of minimally invasive surgical procedures. Each facet of care, including preoperative preparation, appropriate patient positioning, trocar placement, and surgical technique, is reviewed, and recommendations are made to facilitate the performance of safe surgery and immediate recognition of complications if they do arise.

**Abdominal Wall Endometriosis**                                                    369

Christine E. Foley, Patricia Giglio Ayers, and Ted T. Lee

> Abdominal wall endometriosis (AWE) is a rare type of endometriosis defined as endometrial glands and stroma located within the abdominal wall. Patients with a history of prior abdominal surgery classically present with cyclic abdominal pain and a palpable mass. Definitive diagnosis is made by pathologic tissue examination, but preoperative imaging with ultrasonography or MRI helps narrow the differential and informs surgical management. Surgical management is traditionally via an open approach; however, laparoscopic removal of AWE is recommended for subfascial or rectus lesions. Following surgical excision, more than 90% of patients experience complete symptom relief.

**Enhanced Recovery After Surgery in Minimally Invasive Gynecologic Surgery**        381

Lisa Chao, Emily Lin, and Kimberly Kho

> Enhanced recovery after surgery (ERAS) is a multimodal, multidisciplinary approach to optimize patient outcomes by minimizing surgical stress with the goal of returning to normal physiologic function. Using minimally invasive surgery as the preferred route for gynecologic surgery is an integral component of ERAS and is strongly correlated with improved postoperative outcomes. Implementation of ERAS programs in minimally invasive gynecologic surgery results in substantial improvements in clinical outcomes with higher rates of same-day discharge, reduction in postoperative nausea and vomiting, improved patient satisfaction, and decreased opioid consumption without increase in complications, readmissions, or health care costs.

# OBSTETRICS AND GYNECOLOGY CLINICS

**FORTHCOMING ISSUES**

*September 2022*
**Emergencies in Obstetrics and Gynecology**
Patricia S. Huguelet and Henry L. Galan, *Editors*

*December 2022*
**Global Women's Health**
Jean R. Anderson and Grace Chen, *Editors*

*March 2023*
**Drugs in Pregnancy**
Catherine Stika, *Editor*

**RECENT ISSUES**

*March 2022*
**Management of Benign and Malignant Breast Disease**
Jessica F. Partin and Patrice M. Weiss, *Editors*

*December 2021*
**A Vision of the Future of Obstetrics and Gynecology**
Denisse S. Holcomb and F. Garry Cunningham, *Editors*

*September 2021*
**Advances in Urogynecology**
Heidi Wendell Brown and Rebecca G. Rogers, *Editors*

**SERIES OF RELATED INTEREST**

*Clinics in Perinatology*
www.perinatology.theclinics.com
*Pediatric Clinics of North America*
https://www.pediatrics.theclinics.com

**THE CLINICS ARE AVAILABLE ONLINE!**
Access your subscription at:
www.theclinics.com

# Foreword

# Minimally Invasive Gynecologic Surgery: Improving Outcomes and Recovery While Reducing Discomfort and Cost

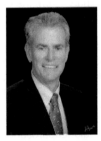

William F. Rayburn, MD, MBA
*Consulting Editor*

This long-awaited issue is the first in *Obstetrics and Gynecology Clinics in North America* to provide an overview of topics pertaining to minimally invasive surgery that apply to gynecologic surgeons. As dual editors, Dr Ted Lee and Dr Nicole Donnellan from the University of Pittsburgh set forth pathways for the reader to diagnose and treat many benign gynecologic disorders. Approaches to chronic pelvic pain, endometriosis, ovarian cysts, myomas, menstrual abnormalities, cervical incompetency, and uterine fibroids are described holistically, that is, more than merely the sum of its parts.

Surgeries described in this issue are to be selected based on their likelihood of improving outcomes due to the complexity of the case or patient factors, with appropriate consideration to costs. Choosing the appropriate patient and counseling about procedural options are essential. For every gynecologic condition described in each article, the authors begin with diagnostic modalities and patient education to assist in the surgical planning. Individualized plans might involve any of the following minimally invasive procedures: hysteroscopy, laparoscopy, robotic surgery, and vaginal surgery. Informed consent should be obtained from patients before surgery with a discussion of the gynecologist's experience, indication(s) for surgery, and potential risks and benefits.

Minimally invasive surgery involves several techniques to operate with less damage to the body than with open abdominal surgery. Anticipated intraoperative and postoperative complications, operative and recovery times, and discomfort with each

https://doi.org/10.1016/j.ogc.2022.04.002
0889-8545/22/© 2022 Published by Elsevier Inc.
obgyn.theclinics.com

procedure should be compared with alternative approaches. In general, minimally invasive gynecologic surgery (MIGS) is associated with less pain, a shorter stay if hospitalization is even necessary, a shorter recovery time, and fewer complications. As described and illustrated in these pages, surgery is performed through one or more small incisions using small tubes, tiny cameras, and surgical instruments. Whether it be laparoscopic, robotic, or hysteroscopic, MIGS provides a magnified, often 3D view of the surgical site, and aids the gynecologist to operate with precision.

The reader's attention is placed throughout these review articles about recovery after minimally invasive surgery. The concluding article deals with enhanced recovery after surgery (ERAS), which refers to multimodal perioperative care pathways or protocols designed to achieve early recovery. In addition to protocols, key factors to a successful ERAS implementation program involve a multidisciplinary team, the organizational will to change practice, and a real-time system for compliance/outcome auditing.

Credentialing and privileging to perform minimally invasive surgery are conducted locally by heath care institutions, whereas the American Board of Obstetrics and Gynecology provides certification after completion of either resident training or MIGS fellowship training. Medical specialty organizations, other educational institutions, and the health care industry do not have the authority to credential or privilege but may provide documented training for gynecologists. Some medical specialty organizations, such as the American Association of Gynecologic Laparoscopists, have developed guidelines for credentialing and privileging to use as templates and modified for each individual institution.

Content in this issue should serve as a valuable resource for gynecologic surgeons at any level. Dr Lee and Dr Donnellan gathered a team of experts who provide practical approaches and many technical "pearls" for a contemporary, holistic, and patient-centered focus. The authors share their knowledge about the technology and multitude of treatment options for meaningful decision making shared between the patient and surgeon. I look forward to an update that reflects the expansion of a rapidly growing literature that reports.

William F. Rayburn, MD, MBA
Department of Obstetrics and Gynecology
Medical University of South Carolina
1721 Atlantic Avenue
Sullivan's Island, SC 294482, USA

E-mail address:
wrayburnmd@gmail.com

# Preface

# Holistic Approach to Minimally Invasive Gynecologic Surgery

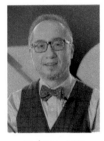
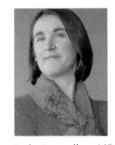

Ted Lee, MD    Nicole Donnellan, MD
*Editors*

When we were invited to be editors for this issue of *Obstetrics and Gynecology Clinics of North America* on minimally invasive gynecologic surgery, we decided to create content that can enhance the practice of generalists and specialists alike. While there are plenty of technical pearls offered by our team of experts throughout the following pages, the articles were thoughtfully compiled to provide the most up-to-date, holistic, patient-centered approach to minimally invasive gynecologic surgery, which we believe is the key to optimizing patient outcomes.

The success of a surgery starts long before the procedure itself. Understanding accurate diagnostic modalities that will assist in surgical planning and the informed consent process is paramount to optimizing surgical outcomes, as is evident in the articles on abdominal wall endometriosis and cerclage. Recognizing such conditions and having knowledge of minimally invasive options available play an important role in providing patient-centered care in minimally invasive gynecologic surgery. Once surgery is decided upon, working with anesthesia colleagues to develop enhanced recovery after surgery ("ERAS") allows surgeons to focus on subtle details in perioperative planning that can dramatically alter the patient's perception of the surgery and overall satisfaction of the episode of care.

Taking a holistic approach to patient care is especially crucial for many of our patients with pelvic pain. The role of hysterectomy, with appropriate patient selection and counseling, may be a surgical option, as discussed by Tu and colleagues. A highly skilled surgeon with impeccable techniques can perform hysterectomy or fertility-sparing surgery; however, it takes a village to ensure comprehensive evaluation and management of chronic pelvic pain. The team from Michigan addresses the importance of recognizing and managing coexisting overlapping pain conditions in the comprehensive care of pelvic pain.

Obstet Gynecol Clin N Am 49 (2022) xv–xvi
https://doi.org/10.1016/j.ogc.2022.04.001
0889-8545/22/© 2022 Published by Elsevier Inc.    obgyn.theclinics.com

Shared decision making is a key component of patient-centered health care. It is important for providers to be knowledgeable about the evolving technology and the multitude of treatment options to inform meaningful shared decision making. The articles on fibroids as well as the reviews on robotic surgery and office-based hysteroscopy provide exactly the type of information to assist providers and patients in making meaningful decisions in their own care. The article on practical approach to fertility considerations in endometriosis surgery epitomizes shared decision making, with well-delineated, evidence-based benefits and harms of common clinical scenarios.

Complications are an inevitable part of surgery, and we would be remiss to not include an article on the importance of early recognition and management of common complications following minimally invasive gynecologic surgery.

We truly appreciate the time and effort our panel of experts dedicated to this special issue. The content provided in the subsequent articles will serve as an invaluable resource for gynecologists to elevate the care of our patients for years to come.

Ted Lee, MD
Minimally Invasive Gynecologic Surgery
Department of OB/GYN/RS
University of Pittsburgh School of Medicine
Magee Womens Hospital of UPMC
Pittsburgh, PA 15213, USA

Nicole Donnellan, MD
OB/GYN/RS Residency
FMIGS
Department of OB/GYN/RS
University of Pittsburgh School of Medicine
Magee-Womens Hospital of UPMC
Pittsburgh, PA 15213, USA

*E-mail addresses:*
leextt@upmc.edu (T. Lee)
donnellann2@upmc.edu (N. Donnellan)

# Approach to Diagnosis and Management of Chronic Pelvic Pain in Women

## Incorporating Chronic Overlapping Pain Conditions in Assessment and Management

Sara R. Till, MD, MPH[a],*, Reina Nakamura, DO[b],
Andrew Schrepf, PhD[c], Sawsan As-Sanie, MD, MPH[a]

## KEYWORDS

• Endometriosis • Vulvodynia • Pelvic myofascial pain • Central sensitization

## KEY POINTS

• Half of the patients with chronic pelvic pain (CPP) have nongynecologic conditions contributing to pain symptoms.
• Patients with gynecologic pain conditions, such as endometriosis and vulvodynia, may be more vulnerable to the development of additional chronic overlapping pain conditions (COPCs).
• Pelvic myofascial pain should be considered in patients who suffer from gynecologic or pelvic COPCs, including endometriosis, vulvodynia, interstitial cystitis/bladder pain syndrome, or irritable bowel syndrome.
• Patients and clinicians should be aware that patients with multiple COPCs and higher degrees of central sensitization may not experience as robust an improvement with peripheral strategies alone.

## INTRODUCTION

At least 15% to 20% of women suffer from chronic pelvic pain, which is defined as pain occurring in the abdomen or pelvis for at least 14 days per month and is severe enough to cause functional limitations or prompt medical care.[1] This condition has a profound impact on physical health, emotional well-being, and ability to function

[a] Department of Obstetrics and Gynecology, University of Michigan, 1500 East Medical Center Drive, Ann Arbor, MI 48109, USA; [b] Department of Physical Medicine and Rehabilitation, University of Michigan, 325 East Eisenhower Parkway, Ann Arbor, MI 48108, USA; [c] Department of Anesthesiology, University of Michigan, 24 Frank Lloyd Wright Drive, Ann Arbor, MI 48105, USA
* Corresponding author.
*E-mail address:* tillsa@med.umich.edu

Obstet Gynecol Clin N Am 49 (2022) 219–239
https://doi.org/10.1016/j.ogc.2022.02.006
0889-8545/22/© 2022 Elsevier Inc. All rights reserved.

across family, social, and professional roles. Chronic pelvic pain is notoriously challenging to manage, frustrating patients and clinicians alike.

One of the reasons that chronic pelvic pain is so difficult to treat is that it is both multifactorial in etiology and highly heterogeneous in presentation. Although gynecologic etiologies, such as endometriosis, are commonly identified in patients with chronic pelvic pain, about half of patients with chronic pelvic pain have nongynecologic conditions contributing to their symptoms.[2] Patients with chronic pelvic pain very frequently suffer from other nonpelvic pain conditions, particularly those that comprise the chronic overlapping pain conditions (COPCs). COPCs are a set of chronic pain conditions that have a high probability of co-occurrence and appear to share common underlying mechanisms and risk factors. Two gynecologic pain conditions are included in the National Institutes of Health Pain Consortium list of COPCs: endometriosis and vulvodynia. But COPCs also include both pelvic (interstitial cystitis/bladder pain syndrome [IC/BPS] and irritable bowel syndrome [IBS]) and nonpelvic conditions (fibromyalgia, temporomandibular disorders [TMDs], migraine headache, chronic tension-type headache, chronic low back pain, and myalgic encephalomyelitis/chronic fatigue syndrome [ME/CFS]). The conditions that contribute to chronic pelvic pain symptoms in one person often differ greatly from those that contribute in another and can change in any given patient over their life course.

The presence of persistent pain, regardless of specific cause or location, can lead to increased sensitization of the central nervous system—in other words, predisposing patients to the development of additional chronic pain conditions.[3,4] Notably, patients with multiple chronic pain conditions often respond less robustly to treatments focused on individual conditions.[5–7] Therefore, it is essential to approach the management of chronic pelvic pain in a comprehensive manner, which includes identification of all conditions that contribute to pain symptoms and optimal management of each contributing condition.

The objectives of this review are to briefly review gynecologic, pelvic, and nonpelvic pain conditions that frequently occur in patients with chronic pelvic pain, to discuss how the presence of these overlapping conditions may influence treatment response, and to review some general management strategies for chronic pelvic pain, with particular attention to patients with co-occurring COPCs.

## BRIEF REVIEW OF INDIVIDUAL CHRONIC OVERLAPPING PAIN CONDITIONS

In this section, we briefly review individual COPCs with the goal of familiarizing clinicians with these disorders so that they are more likely to recognize co-occurring conditions outside of their clinical expertise. We have organized this discussion by gynecologic, pelvic, and nonpelvic conditions. This is certainly not a comprehensive list of all potential conditions that may contribute to pain symptoms. For example, many patients with pelvic pain have significant contributions from pelvic myofascial pain, which we have discussed in detail in the Evaluation section below. Rather, this section is intended to serve as a brief introduction to this defined category of COPCs that are often underdiagnosed in patients with chronic pain, with the goal of facilitating screening and prompting referral to appropriate specialists.

### Gynecologic Pain Conditions

#### Endometriosis
Endometriosis is a condition in which endometrial-like tissue is present outside the uterus. It is estimated to affect 10% of women of reproductive age.[8] Prevalence is much higher in women presenting with chronic pelvic pain (over 70%)[9] and in those

with infertility (21%–47%).[10] Endometriosis is most commonly found on the pelvic peritoneum, ovaries, tubes, but can also grow on other pelvic structures, such as colon, bladder, or appendix, and in more distant sites, such as diaphragm or pleural space. Endometriosis is classified according to stages using a variety of classification systems (eg, ASRM, Enzian, AAGL), all of which represent the anatomic disease burden identified at the time of surgical exploration. Although the higher stage corresponds to a higher probability of fertility-related issues and surgical complexity, it has little if any correlation with the degree of pain symptoms except dyspareunia.[11–13]

Symptoms of endometriosis are highly variable but may include dysmenorrhea, noncyclic pelvic pain, dyspareunia, dysuria, dyschezia, or infertility. Diagnosis of endometriosis is inherently challenging due to lack of reliable noninvasive diagnostic tools, heterogeneous symptom presentation, and the fact that the associated symptoms are nonspecific and can be seen in a variety of conditions. Although endometriosis may be suspected based on symptoms, diagnosis has traditionally required surgical confirmation. MRI is the most sensitive noninvasive diagnostic modality but is most effective in identifying advanced endometriosis with deep infiltrating lesions or endometriomas and typically does not identify superficial endometriosis lesions. Lack of sensitivity for superficial disease is notable, given high cost associated with MRI.

A recent study examining COPCs in a large health system administrative database evaluated co-occurrence of other COPCs diagnoses based on the index COPC diagnosis. Risk for co-occurrence of COPCs was substantially higher than risk for co-occurrence of several chronic non-pain conditions. For example, patients presenting with endometriosis were most likely to carry diagnoses of IC/BPS (odds ratio [OR] 18.62), vulvodynia (OR 15.56), and IBS (OR 5.05)[14] (**Table 1**).

### Vulvodynia

Vulvodynia is defined as persistent vulvar pain present for at least 3 months without another identifiable etiology.[15] Prevalence is difficult to estimate as the diagnostic criteria have changed in recent years, but is thought to be present in at least 7% of women.[16] Vulvodynia can be spontaneous, provoked by contact, or mixed, and frequently contributes significantly to dyspareunia. Vulvodynia is a diagnosis of exclusion and it is essential to rule out infectious, inflammatory, malignant, and other etiologies before confirming the diagnosis.[15]

### Nongynecologic Pelvic Pain Conditions

### Interstitial cystitis/bladder pain syndrome

IC/BPS is a condition in which patients experience bladder discomfort, most commonly pain but may report primarily pressure or spasm symptoms. Typically, patients report increased discomfort with bladder filling, which improves after bladder emptying. Many patients experience urinary urgency and frequency, which is thought to be a coping technique to avoid the discomfort associated with bladder distention. This constellation of symptoms is frequently interpreted by patients and health care providers as a urinary tract infection, but typically patients will have an unremarkable urinalysis or urine culture.

Diagnosis of IC/BPS has evolved substantially over the last few decades. Current diagnostic criteria focus primarily on clinical symptoms. Additional testing, including urinalysis, urodynamics, cystoscopy, is used selectively to exclude other conditions that may have a similar presentation.[17] Selective cystoscopy is currently recommended to rule out other etiologies, such as malignancy or foreign body, in patients who are high-risk, or who are nonresponsive to conservative therapy.[18] Both the evolution

**Table 1**
Odd ratios for pairs of COPCs and three chronic non-COPCs with 95% confidence intervals

| | FM | | | JBS | | | TMO | | | UCPPS | | | ENDO | | |
|---|---|---|---|---|---|---|---|---|---|---|---|---|---|---|---|
| | OR | LL | UL | OR | LL | UL | OR | LL | UL | OR | LL | UL | OR | LL | UL |
| FM | | | | 10.18 | 9.72 | 10.67 | 5.64 | 4.98 | 6.40 | 9.91 | 8.88 | 11.06 | 4.06 | 3.49 | 4.72 |
| IBS | 10.18 | 9.72 | 10.67 | | | | 3.70 | 3.27 | 4.18 | 9.10 | 8.27 | 10.02 | 5.05 | 4.46 | 5.72 |
| TMD | 5.64 | 4.98 | 6.40 | 3.70 | 3.27 | 4.18 | | | | 4.75 | 3.61 | 6.25 | 1.87 | 1.22 | 2.89 |
| UCPPS | 9.91 | 8.88 | 11.06 | 9.10 | 8.27 | 10.02 | 4.75 | 3.61 | 6.25 | | | | 18.62 | 15.74 | 22.03 |
| ENDO | 4.06 | 3.49 | 4.72 | 5.05 | 4.46 | 5.72 | 1.87 | 1.22 | 2.89 | 18.62 | 15.74 | 22.03 | | | |
| VVD | 3.14 | 2.65 | 3.73 | 3.97 | 3.46 | 4.56 | 1.85 | 1.19 | 2.88 | 24.99 | 21.41 | 29.16 | 15.56 | 12.77 | 18.95 |
| cLBP | 5.29 | 5.09 | 5.51 | 2.29 | 2.20 | 2.39 | 1.24 | 1.10 | 1.40 | 2.34 | 2.11 | 2.60 | 2.30 | 2.04 | 2.60 |
| cTTH | 2.43 | 2.10 | 2.81 | 1.58 | 1.37 | 1.82 | 2.64 | 2.01 | 3.47 | 1.94 | 1.38 | 2.72 | 1.25 | 0.79 | 1.97 |
| MHA | 5.27 | 5.06 | 5.50 | 3.30 | 3.18 | 3.43 | 6.13 | 5.66 | 6.64 | 3.29 | 2.98 | 3.64 | 3.21 | 2.88 | 3.58 |
| CFS | 6.07 | 5.64 | 6.52 | 2.90 | 2.68 | 3.14 | 1.48 | 1.14 | 1.91 | 2.78 | 2.27 | 3.42 | 1.86 | 1.43 | 2.43 |
| DN | 2.60 | 2.27 | 2.98 | 1.66 | 1.45 | 1.90 | N/A | N/A | N/A | 0.86 | 0.52 | 1.40 | N/A | N/A | N/A |
| COPD | 3.14 | 2.94 | 3.36 | 1.78 | 1.66 | 1.90 | 0.89 | 0.71 | 1.12 | 1.05 | 0.84 | 1.31 | 0.54 | 0.37 | 0.80 |
| CVH | 2.20 | 1.88 | 2.57 | 1.48 | 1.27 | 1.72 | 0.56 | 0.31 | 1.02 | 1.19 | 0.76 | 1.84 | N/A | N/A | N/A |

| | VVD | | | cLBP | | | cTTH | | | MHA | | | ME/CFS | | |
|---|---|---|---|---|---|---|---|---|---|---|---|---|---|---|---|
| | OR | LL | UL | OR | LL | UL | OR | LL | UL | OR | LL | UL | OR | LL | UL |
| FM | 3.14 | 2.65 | 3.73 | 5.29 | 5.09 | 5.51 | 2.43 | 2.10 | 2.81 | 5.27 | 5.06 | 5.50 | 6.07 | 5.64 | 6.52 |
| IBS | 3.97 | 3.46 | 4.56 | 2.29 | 2.20 | 2.39 | 1.58 | 1.37 | 1.82 | 3.30 | 3.18 | 3.43 | 2.90 | 2.68 | 3.14 |
| TMO | 1.85 | 1.19 | 2.88 | 1.24 | 1.10 | 1.40 | 2.64 | 2.01 | 3.47 | 6.13 | 5.66 | 6.64 | 1.48 | 1.14 | 1.91 |
| UCPPS | 24.99 | 21.41 | 29.16 | 2.34 | 2.11 | 2.60 | 1.94 | 1.38 | 2.72 | 3.29 | 2.98 | 3.64 | 2.78 | 2.27 | 3.42 |
| ENDO | 15.56 | 12.77 | 18.95 | 2.30 | 2.04 | 2.60 | 1.25 | 0.79 | 1.97 | 3.21 | 2.88 | 3.58 | 1.86 | 1.43 | 2.43 |
| VVD | | | | 1.20 | 1.02 | 1.40 | N/A | N/A | N/A | 1.63 | 1.42 | 1.87 | 1.19 | 0.85 | 1.66 |
| cLBP | 1.20 | 1.02 | 1.40 | | | | 1.26 | 1.15 | 1.39 | 1.99 | 1.93 | 2.05 | 1.75 | 1.65 | 1.86 |
| cTTH | N/A | N/A | N/A | 1.26 | 1.15 | 1.39 | | | | 4.27 | 3.98 | 4.58 | 1.82 | 1.51 | 2.20 |
| MHA | 1.63 | 1.42 | 1.87 | 1.99 | 1.93 | 2.05 | 4.27 | 3.98 | 4.58 | | | | 2.67 | 2.52 | 2.83 |

| | | | | | | | | | | | | | | | |
|---|---|---|---|---|---|---|---|---|---|---|---|---|---|---|---|
| ME/CFS | 1.19 | 0.85 | 1.66 | 1.75 | 1.65 | 1.86 | 1.82 | 1.51 | 2.20 | 2.67 | 2.52 | 2.83 | | | |
| DN | N/A | N/A | N/A | 2.08 | 1.93 | 2.26 | 0.51 | 0.32 | 0.82 | 1.06 | 0.95 | 1.19 | 1.18 | 0.94 | 1.48 |
| COPD | 0.50 | 0.33 | 0.75 | 1.92 | 1.84 | 2.00 | 0.71 | 0.58 | 0.87 | 1.11 | 1.05 | 1.17 | 1.29 | 1.16 | 1.44 |
| CVH | N/A | N/A | N/A | 1.22 | 1.10 | 1.35 | 0.56 | 0.35 | 0.91 | 0.68 | 0.59 | 0.78 | 1.01 | 0.79 | 1.31 |
| | | | | | | 0–1 | 1–3 | 2–5 | 5+ | | | | | | |

Colors correspond to the strength of the relationship: light blue = moderate negative relationship; light yellow = moderate positive relationship; orange = strong positive relationship; and red = very strong positive relationship.

*Abbreviations:* cLBP, chronic low back pain; COPD, chronic obstructive pulmonary disease; cTTH, chronic tension-type headache; CVH, chronic viral hepatitis; DN, diabetic neuropathy; ENDO, endometriosis; FM, fibromyalgia; IBS, irritable bowel syndrome; ME/CFS, myalgic encephalomyelitis/chronic fatigue syndrome; MHA, migraine headache; TMD, temporomandibular disorder; UCPPS, urologic chronic pelvic pain syndrome; VVD, vulvodynia.

*From* Schrepf A, Phan V, Clemens JQ, Maixner W, Hanauer D, Williams DA. ICD-10 Codes for the Study of Chronic Overlapping Pain Conditions in Administrative Databases. J Pain. 2020;21(1-2):59-70. https://doi.org/10.1016/j.jpain.2019.05.007; with permission.

of diagnostic criteria and the fact that IC/BPS is essentially a diagnosis of exclusion complicates estimates of prevalence. The most comprehensive assessments to date indicate 2% to 6% prevalence.[19] There is a very high prevalence of tenderness to palpation of bladder, urethra, and pelvic floor, indicating that pelvic myofascial pain is likely a significant contributor for many patients with this condition.

### Irritable bowel syndrome

IBS is a functional gastrointestinal condition in which patients experience chronic abdominal pain and altered bowel habits. Abdominal pain symptoms may be intermittent or persistent, are often associated with bloating and increased gas production, and are frequently exacerbated with defecation. Patients may report diarrhea, constipation, or alternating stool consistency.[20] Prevalence of IBS is estimated to be around 11%, but fewer than half of patients have received a formal diagnosis by many estimates.[21] Diagnosis of IBS is primarily clinical, but evaluation should include at least a limited assessment to exclude other gastrointestinal conditions such as inflammatory bowel disease or structural lesions. For example, colonoscopy may be recommended if patients present with diarrhea and other alarming features, such as weight loss or onset of symptoms after age 50 years. Abdominal computed tomography scan may be recommended in patients who present with persistent constipation along with early satiety, pain, and bloating.

## Nonpelvic Pain Conditions

### Migraine headache

Migraine headache is a debilitating condition that is the third most prevalent condition in the world and the seventh leading cause of global burden of disease, affecting more than 10% of the world's population.[22] The 2 major subtypes are migraine without aura and migraine with aura. Migraine without aura is described as a moderate to severe unilateral pulsatile headache aggravated by physical activity and lasts 4 to 72 hours.[22] Many patients also experience nausea/vomiting, photophobia, and/or phonophobia. Migraine with aura is characterized by headache with preceding or accompanying transient focal neurologic symptoms. Typically, these episodes include visual or other sensory manifestations that are brief (minutes), unilateral, and fully reversible.[22]

### Chronic tension-type headache

Chronic tension-type headache is defined as nonthrobbing headache present for at least 15 days per month for at least 6-month duration. Pain is much more likely to be present bilaterally compared to migraine but can occur unilaterally. Patients typically describe symptoms as pressure, squeezing, tightening, or "band-like." Tension-type headache is extremely common, estimated between 40% and 80% prevalence, but is episodic in the vast majority of cases.[23] Prevalence of chronic tension-type headache is estimated around 1% to 2%.[23] Migraine headache and chronic tension-type headache are not mutually exclusive and it is common for patients to suffer from both.

### Temporomandibular disorders

TMDs are a group of musculoskeletal and neuromuscular disorders affecting the temporomandibular joint, muscles of mastication, and/or surrounding soft tissues.[24] Symptoms include dull, unilateral facial pain that is typically constant with intermittent exacerbations, often provoked by jaw motion. Pain often radiates toward the neck, ear, temporal, or periorbital areas. The prevalence of TMD is estimated to be at least 6% and is nearly twice as common among women than men.[25]

*Chronic low back pain*
Chronic low back pain is defined as back pain that continues for at least 12 weeks. Pain symptoms are variable, ranging from dull and aching to sharp and shooting. Most episodes of low back pain are self-limited and resolve within a few days to weeks. But approximately 20% of people with acute low back pain will develop more persistent symptoms. Although acute low back pain is extremely common, the prevalence of chronic low back pain is thought to be between 8% and 10%.[26] Etiology of low back pain is highly variable and may include myofascial, nerve, or bony contributions. Risk factors include increasing age, obesity, poor fitness level, and occupational factors, among others.

*Fibromyalgia*
Fibromyalgia is characterized by chronic widespread pain, fatigue, sleep disturbance, mood changes, and somatic symptoms.[27] Prevalence is estimated between 2% and 8%.[27] Central sensitization, or nociplastic pain, appears to play an important role in this condition.[27,28] Because the pain associated with fibromyalgia is widespread, it can be challenging to rule out other conditions, such as autoimmune disorders or osteoarthritis. Diagnosis is typically made by clinical history and physical examination, and imaging and laboratory studies are typically not useful except for ruling out other suspected diagnoses.[27] For example, pain limited to joints or pain associated with swelling of joints should prompt evaluation for an autoimmune condition such as rheumatoid arthritis. It is essential to note that this is not a disorder of the central nervous system alone and most patients with fibromyalgia have peripheral pain contributors, such as degenerative disc disease or osteoarthritis. However, patients with fibromyalgia typically perceive a greater degree of pain than would otherwise be anticipated based on the peripheral or nociceptive input.[29]

*Myalgic encephalomyelitis/chronic fatigue syndrome*
ME/CFS is characterized by at least 6-month duration of moderate to severe fatigue occurring at least 50% of the time, which is not relieved by rest, and is associated with symptoms such as postexertional malaise, sleep disturbance, cognitive dysfunction, pain, and orthostatic symptoms.[30] The prevalence is also variable due to multiple definitions of ME/CFS. Although the point prevalence of chronic fatigue seems to be at least 2% to 6%, the prevalence of patients meeting full diagnostic criteria for ME/CFS is likely less than 0.5%.[31,32]

## RISK FACTORS FOR CHRONIC PAIN CONDITIONS

Studies examining risk factors for the development of chronic pain are abundant, and yet our understanding of the true underlying mechanisms that correspond to these risk factors remains limited. For example, many studies have demonstrated a relationship between chronic pain conditions and low socioeconomic status, lower educational attainment, unemployment, poor nutrition, limited physical activity, obesity, sleep disorders, mental health conditions, tobacco use, alcohol use, and opioid use.[33,34] But one can certainly understand the bidirectional relationship associated with these factors—experiencing chronic pain predisposes to the development of all of these issues. Similarly, it is challenging to disentangle the influence of age, race, sex, and history of abuse or trauma from factors such as health care provider unconscious bias or patient willingness to report pain symptoms, particularly relative to pain diagnoses that are associated more with functional than overtly anatomic etiologies.

   With those caveats, we will focus primarily on 2 risk factors for chronic pain conditions: presence of another chronic pain condition and genetic vulnerability.

The presence of chronic pain in one location more than doubles the risk for development of new chronic pain in other, even distant, locations.[3,35] In fact, in longitudinal studies, the presence of pain in more than one region at baseline was the strongest predictor for development of chronic pain in addition locations.[4] The predisposition to development of additional chronic pain conditions likely relates to altered function in sensory and pain processing pathways in the central nervous system, which is discussed in more detail in the following.

Chronic pelvic pain conditions, such as endometriosis, and COPCs appear to have a significant genetic or heritable vulnerability. Risk for endometriosis increases 7 to 10 fold if present in a first-degree relative and several genetic variants have been identified that appear to be highly consistent with development of endometriosis as well as severity of disease stage.[8,36] There is also evidence of heritable risk for other COPCs based on twin studies. A large twin study of over 31,000 participants in Sweden indicated that a latent genetic risk factor was associated with all 4 of the COPCs under investigation (recurrent headache, IBS, ME/CFS, and chronic widespread pain).[37] Similarly, first-degree relatives of patients with a COPC appear to be more likely to have diverse pain manifestations, not only the COPC under investigation but these associations may also be due to shared environmental risk.[38,39]

## COMMON MECHANISMS IN CHRONIC PAIN CONDITIONS

A growing body of evidence supports the concept that there are shared risk factors and pathophysiological mechanisms in the appearance of chronic pelvic pain and COPCs. Central sensitization, central pain amplification, and nociplastic pain are 3 terms with considerable overlap and all describe central nervous system abnormalities in sensory and pain processing pathways that ultimately augment and maintain chronic pain. A recent review covers these mechanisms in detail,[40] so we will only briefly summarize that literature here. Functional, structural, and chemical neuroimaging studies have demonstrated differences between patients with COPCs and healthy controls in resting-state connectivity, gray matter volume, and levels of excitatory neurotransmitter in sensory regions of the brain.[40] Similarly, many studies have indicated that those with COPCs display heightened sensitivity to experimental pain in areas of the body not considered symptomatic of the COPC—for example, a substantial number of patients with TMD are more sensitive to pain in areas distal from the face and jaw, suggesting a global rather than local pattern of pain sensitivity. This pattern has been noted across several chronic pelvic pain conditions and COPCs, including endometriosis, vulvodynia, IC/BPS, IBS, fibromyalgia, and headache.[41–46] Together, these findings suggest that central nervous system alterations with accompanying global hyperalgesia are generic, rather than condition-specific, features of COPCs. In addition, sensory sensitivity, both to bodily sensations and environmental stimuli, as well as constitutional symptoms such as sleep disturbances, fatigue, and cognitive dysfunction, are common across COPCs.[47,48]

A heightened inflammatory response to ex vivo stimulation of monocytes, t-cells, or whole blood by immunogenic substances is emerging as a marker of COPCs in several conditions. Animal models have consistently demonstrated a role for toll-like receptors (TLRs) in the spinal cord and brain toward pain sensitization and the transition from acute to chronic pain.[49] Studies in pain patients now suggest that the TLR responsiveness in circulating immune cells or whole blood show demonstrate a similar phenomenon. A heightened inflammatory response to lipopolysaccharide, a classic agonist of TLR-4, distinguishes female IC/BPS patients with additional COPCs from those who have pelvic pain only and several other pain conditions including IBS and dysmenorrhea from healthy controls.[50–53]

These findings taken together provide substantial support for neurobiological substrates promoting generic risk for a COPC—the biological evidence for why COPCs do indeed overlap. Of course, additional condition-specific neurobiological risk factors remain an important area for investigation, but disease models that ignore shared biological pathways are necessarily limited to the subset of patients, more exception than rule, who have a single COPC.

Because COPCs share common mechanisms, many of the treatment strategies aimed at these mechanisms may be broadly applicable across many chronic pain conditions. We summarize strategies that target central sensitization in the following section. However, it is worth noting that most patients require multimodal treatment that addresses both the disease-specific or peripheral mechanisms in addition to central sensitization.

## MANAGEMENT STRATEGIES FOR PATIENTS WITH CHRONIC PELVIC PAIN
### Evaluation

A thoughtful and comprehensive history is essential for the evaluation of patients who present with chronic pelvic pain. Evaluation is typically specific to the suspected condition. A thoughtful physical examination and limited use of basic diagnostic or radiologic testing is typically adequate to diagnose many chronic pain conditions. But other conditions require more invasive testing to confirm diagnosis, such as surgical evaluation to confirm endometriosis. In patients with chronic pelvic pain, it is essential to evaluate for pelvic floor myofascial pain and co-occurring COPCs.

### Pelvic myofascial pain
Pelvic myofascial pain is a condition in which pain originates from hypertonic or hypercontractile muscles. Myofascial pain is very common across many chronic pain conditions. Among women with chronic pelvic pain, 60% to 90% have musculoskeletal dysfunction contributing to their pain symptoms.[54,55] Although myofascial pain affects such a large proportion of people with pelvic pain, it is one of the most overlooked diagnoses in this population. Most people with conditions like endometriosis, vulvodynia, IBS, or IC/BPS have some component of myofascial pelvic pain. Pelvic myofascial pain is typically diagnosed based on pain with palpation of pelvic floor muscles, typically accessed through the vagina.

Symptoms of myofascial pain can vary depending on which muscles are malfunctioning and on the degree of spasticity. Pelvic myofascial pain is typically described as pelvic cramping, pressure, heaviness, aching, throbbing, soreness, or often as a "falling out sensation". Patients often report that pain occurs in the pelvis, vagina, vulva, bladder, or rectum, but frequently radiates to hips, buttocks, or legs. Pain often worsens throughout the day or with activities, such as standing or driving for long periods. Many people have exacerbations of pain related to menstrual periods, intercourse, bowel movements, urination, or having a full bladder, and pain can last for hours or days after an aggravating episode.

It is important to note that there is often overlap between symptoms of myofascial pelvic pain and other pelvic pain conditions, like endometriosis, vulvodynia, IBS, and bladder pain syndrome. Because the pelvic floor muscles are connected to and support the function of the pelvic organs, and because the pelvic floor muscles and pelvic organs share many sensory nerve pathways, it can be challenging to distinguish between pain originating in the pelvic organs versus the muscles based on symptoms alone.

### Co-occurring chronic overlapping pain conditions

Primary care providers are typically more well versed in performing a thorough review of systems and obtaining a full picture of health history, whereas specialists often focus almost exclusively on the condition within their area of expertise. The risk of focused assessment is that a specialist may remain unaware of or may not uncover a patient's other COPCs, particularly given that many patients may not have the condition listed in their electronic medical record or have received a formal diagnosis. As discussed earlier, patients who have multiple COPCs or a significant degree of central sensitization often do not respond as robustly to peripherally focused treatments. So early identification of this risk factor can help the clinician and patient to have a more informed risk-benefit discussion regarding treatment options, particularly those associated with significant risk or recovery time such as surgical procedures.

Although it is not feasible or advisable for a subspecialist to manage conditions outside of their clinical expertise, simple screening measures can identify possible chronic pain conditions and features of central sensitization, which may help to facilitate referral to an appropriate specialist.

A fairly simple screening tool is the Complex Medical Symptoms Inventory (CMSI), which is a 41-item questionnaire designed to screen for cardinal symptoms of most COPCs.[56] Some chronic pain referral clinics opt to have patients complete more precise screening measures, such as Rome criteria for IBS or Pain, Urgency, and Frequency (PUF) score for IC/BPS. This is certainly a reasonable strategy if clinicians have the ability and time to interpret the screening tools accurately, particularly if there is a very high rate of overlap between specific conditions. However, clinicians should avoid giving a patient a definitive diagnosis outside of one's own clinical expertise, as many of these conditions are diagnoses of exclusion. Referral to an appropriate specialist ensures that the patient will have access to necessary evaluation to rule out more threatening etiologies.

As a reminder, the presence of a COPC does not absolve clinicians from performing appropriate evaluations for other anatomic or concerning etiologies. Many patients with COPCs have experienced delayed diagnoses of malignant, infectious, or inflammatory conditions because an appropriate evaluation was deferred due to suspicion that new or altered symptoms were likely attributed to their predisposition for the development of new COPCs.

### Communication and Setting Expectations

Many patients with chronic pelvic pain or COPCs have received explicit or implicit messages from clinicians, friends, or family members that their pain was "all in their head." Many feel that their symptoms are not taken as seriously because these disorders are often not associated with significant anatomic abnormalities. Clear and empathetic communication is essential for developing therapeutic rapport. It is critical for clinicians to allow patients to tell their stories, to validate their symptoms and the impact on quality of life, and to be thoughtful and intentional when discussing the interaction between peripheral and central pain contributions.

Although every clinician and patient are hopeful that a particular treatment may result in complete resolution of pain, a focus on anticipated functional improvements may be more appropriate and realistic. Interestingly, many patients report that their goals are similar—they do not necessarily expect to be pain-free, but rather that they do not want pain to continue to dictate the degree to which they are able to participate in family, social, or professional roles. Patients and clinicians may obtain more insightful information about treatment response by asking the patient to identify a few personal functional goals and track progress relative to these rather than continuing to focus exclusively on pain symptoms. Many patients identify improved sleep and fatigue, ability to play with their children, or fewer days of missed work as goals that are more reflective of their quality of life than a "pain score."

### *Treat Peripheral Contributions*

Perception of any painful stimulus involves a complex interaction between peripheral sensory input and pain perception in both the peripheral and central nervous systems. In any given person with a chronic pain condition, there are varying degrees of peripheral input and central amplification contributing to the experience of pain and the likelihood of responding to a specific treatment. For example, endometriosis lesions can create inflammation that activates peripheral nerve receptors. The nerves carry this signal to the spinal cord and brain (central nervous system). The brain then categorizes the type of sensation, interprets location, and assesses intensity and bother associated with the sensation. The brain has a remarkable ability to "triage" or prioritize signals based on situational context. This triaging function is capable of amplifying or diminishing the brain's perception of pain.

This system typically works smoothly in situations involving acute pain, but chronic pain conditions are much more complex. Chronic pain may result from continued peripheral input, such as inflammation due to endometriosis lesions, from abnormal activation of nerves in the peripheral tissues or spinal cord, or from inappropriate triaging or amplification of pain perception in the central nervous system. Optimal treatment of any chronic pain condition must address both peripheral and central contributions.

Identifying all peripheral contributions is an essential step in developing a comprehensive treatment plan, highlighting again the importance of a thoughtful history and physical examination. For example, most patients with endometriosis, vulvodynia, IC/BPS, and IBS also have pelvic myofascial pain. If clinicians focus exclusively on endometriosis lesions or stool consistency without addressing myofascial contribution, patients are unlikely to experience a robust improvement in overall pain symptoms.

Several recent reviews summarize treatment strategies for individual gynecologic pelvic pain conditions,[57,58] so we will only summarize here. For patients with endometriosis, achievement of amenorrhea often results in significant improvement of pain. Surgical treatment of endometriosis can play an important role, but it is worth noting that identification or excision of endometriosis lesions does not rule out the possibility of other pain contributors, such as pelvic myofascial pain, and surgery alone does not represent a comprehensive evaluation.

Myofascial pain is highly prevalent across COPCs and many patients benefit from physical therapy as part of the treatment plan. In addition, physical therapists frequently incorporate pain education, cognitive behavioral strategies, and motivational interviewing in addition to manual therapy, which makes them an invaluable resource in the comprehensive treatment of both chronic pelvic pain and COPCs.[59]

As discussed previously, many patients with multiple COPCs unfortunately may experience less symptom improvement with individual treatment strategies, particularly those that are peripherally focused.[5-7] This certainly does not mean that patients with central sensitization should not have the opportunity to benefit from evidence-based peripheral treatments, such as medical or surgical treatment of endometriosis. But we would argue that clinicians have an ethical responsibility to include accurate information about anticipated outcomes in informed consent discussions, particularly when the patient is considering more invasive interventions such as surgery.

### Treat Co-occurring Psychological Conditions

Prevalence of psychological conditions, such as depression and anxiety, is substantially increased in patients with chronic pain conditions compared with the general population, between 3- and 5-fold increased prevalence by most estimates.[60–64] Patients with concurrent chronic pain and psychological conditions experience more severe pain and worse quality of life compared with patients with chronic pain alone.[62,65]

Several theories have been proposed to explain the high rate of co-occurrence of chronic pain and psychological conditions, and a recent review addresses these in detail[66] so we will only summarize here. The relationship is almost certainly multifactorial, involving common genetic, inflammatory, and neurobiological vulnerabilities. We do believe that it is critical to highlight recent literature on the temporal relationship between these conditions. Several large prospective cohort studies indicate that pain predisposes to the development of mood disorders to a much greater degree than the reverse,[67,68] indicating that pain is not simply a manifestation of psychological distress.

Thoughtful presentation regarding the relationship between chronic pain and psychological conditions is essential in discussions with patients, as many may have had previous interactions within the medical community in which they felt that their pain was dismissed as psychological in origin and therefore may be quite hesitant to consider treatments targeting "mood disorders."

There are several validated tools that clinicians can use to screen for depression and anxiety. Some of the most widely used are PROMIS depression and PROMIS anxiety, which were developed in conjunction with the NIH as part of a large program to develop highly reliable measurement tools for a variety of patient-reported outcomes.[69] These screening tools are public availably, widely used in clinical practice or research applications, and have both long and short versions as well as Spanish-language versions. The Beck Depression Inventory (BDI) and Beck Anxiety Inventory (BAI) are examples of other widely used, validated screening tools.

Focusing on the fact that we consider pain and psychological conditions to be distinct and separate diagnoses, clarifying our current understanding of the temporal relationship between the two, and highlighting the degree to which co-occurrence negatively impacts well-being and quality of life may help the patient to be more willing to consider treatment. This is likely to be much better received once a clinician has developed rapport and made substantive proposals to address peripheral pain contributions.

Finally, management of psychological conditions is best performed by a clinician who has experience in managing these medications and who can follow patients closely to make appropriate medication adjustments. Developing relationships with local psychiatric providers or primary care providers can help to facilitate timely and appropriate treatment.

### Treat Central Sensitization

There is increasing recognition of the role that central sensitization plays in many chronic pain conditions, but much work remains in terms of screening for individual patients and in developing effective management strategies.

One of the most basic yet instructive screening tools is the American College of Rheumatology (ACR) 2011 Fibromyalgia Survey Score.[70] This self-report screening tool includes 2 components: the widespread pain index, which is the sum of total number of painful areas on a body map (0–19 points), and the symptom severity index, which asks about related symptoms such as fatigue, sleep dysfunction, or cognitive symptoms (0–12 points). A score of $\geq 13$ is diagnostic of fibromyalgia. However, the tool is frequently used as a continuous scale (0–31 points) that corresponds to the degree of central sensitization or nociplastic pain.[71] This measure is well validated for this purpose, has demonstrated excellent reliability, is highly predictive of pain and disability, and strongly corresponds to findings of central sensitization on functional neuroimaging.

Various pharmacologic and nonpharmacologic interventions have been evaluated to manage central sensitization, often with modest or conflicting results. Much of the difficulty is related to substantial heterogeneity among the conditions in which central sensitization contributes significantly. Furthermore, there is substantial heterogeneity with regard to the balance of peripheral and central contributions between individual patients with the same condition. Many chronic pain researchers and clinicians have endorsed a move to develop personalized treatment strategies, in which characteristics of an individual patient help clinicians predict which management strategies are likely to yield the greatest benefit, as opposed to relying on the current "trial and error" method.

Current best practices include using a multimodal approach that combines nonpharmacologic and pharmacologic strategies. Much of the available data for these strategies focus on specific COPCs, but we will focus primarily on strategies that have been used for chronic pelvic pain or are widely applicable for COPCs (**Table 2**).

### Nonpharmacologic strategies

Exercise interventions have been evaluated across a multitude of chronic pain conditions and demonstrate improvements in pain, mood, sleep quality, and physical function.[72–74] Mechanism of action is unknown, but proposed theories include

| Table 2 | |
|---|---|
| **Managing central sensitization** | |
| **Management Strategy** | **Clinical Pearls** |
| Multimodal approach is key | Address peripheral contributors and co-occurring psychological conditions |
| Nonpharmacologic options | |
|   Exercise and physical activity | "Start low, go slow" <br> Yoga, aerobic, resistance |
|   Cognitive behavioral therapy | Focus on functional improvement and coping mechanisms |
|   Acupuncture/Acupressure | Work with local physical therapists and primary care physicians to find reputable and experienced providers |
| Pharmacologic options | |
|   Antidepressants (TCA, SNRI) | Presentation is key—focus on neurotransmitter function rather than mood symptoms |
|   Cyclobenzaprine | Addresses the "chronic pain triad"—myofascial pain, poor sleep, and central sensitization |
|   Gabapentinoids | Use most or all of daily dose at bedtime to reduce daytime sedation |
|   Cannabinoids | Know regulations in your state <br> CBD ± THC <br> Oral has longer duration of benefit than inhaled <br> Topical may be less beneficial |

anti-inflammatory effects, improvements in muscle function, and improved pain tolerance with repeated exposure to low levels of exercise-related discomfort. Many forms of exercise have been studied, including aerobic, resistance, and yoga, and there does not seem to be a clear optimal form. It may be best to encourage the patient to begin with an activity that they enjoy rather than prescribing a particular type of "exercise program." It is recommended to counsel patients to "start low and go slow" in terms of intensity and duration in order to minimize risk for pain exacerbations that may occur with an abrupt increase in activity level.[27]

Cognitive behavioral therapy (CBT) is a form of goal-directed psychological therapy that aims to help patients understand how their thoughts and behaviors may be contributing to their environment or disorder and focuses on tools to help modify those thoughts and behaviors. Pain education is also an integral component of CBT. It is very common for patients to develop maladaptive pain avoidance behaviors when pain has been present for a long time, and CBT can be very beneficial in helping to develop more adaptive coping techniques. Notably, CBT appears to be beneficial even in patients without mood disorders, suggesting broad applicability in the management of chronic pain conditions.[75] CBT has been evaluated in a variety of chronic pain conditions and has been associated with improvement in pain, physical function, and mood symptoms.[76–79] Interestingly, CBT modulated connections in pain-processing regions of the brain on functional MRI in patients with endometriosis.[18,80] Careful presentation of this strategy is essential, as many patients with chronic pain conditions may be hesitant to consider "therapy" given prior experiences with pain being dismissed as psychological in origin. Focus instead on the degree to which chronic pain has impacted physical function, sleep, mood, and relationships, and emphasize the potential for the development of more adaptive coping skills to improve quality of life.

Acupuncture is a traditional Chinese medicine therapy that targets specific points along "meridians" or pathways that run through the body. Acupuncture uses very thin needles to target these points, whereas acupressure uses external manual application of pressure. In dysmenorrhea and endometriosis, acupuncture or acupressure were associated with improvements in pain, physical function, fatigue, and quality of life.[78,81–83] Although many of the available studies are low quality or have high risk for bias, this appears to be a low-risk option when performed by trained providers and many patients anecdotally report success.

### Pharmacologic strategies

Several classes of antidepressants have been used for various chronic pain conditions, particularly tricyclic antidepressants (TCAs) and serotonin–norepinephrine reuptake inhibitors (SNRIs). Both of these classes are thought to decrease pain sensitivity by increasing availability of norepinephrine in the descending pain modulatory pathways. Much of the data for these medications come from fibromyalgia, where SNRIs have demonstrated significant improvement in pain and quality of life, typically with fairly minimal side effects.[84,85] TCAs are associated with less robust improvement and use is more often limited by bothersome side effects.[86] Again, thoughtful presentation is key when discussing this option with patients and it is important to emphasize the role of neurotransmitters in pain signaling and perception.

Cyclobenzaprine is a centrally acting muscle relaxant that is pharmacologically similar to TCAs. Mechanism of action is also thought to be primarily related to increasing central availability of norepinephrine. In patients with fibromyalgia, use was associated with improved pain, sleep, and fatigue.[87,88] Many patients report drowsiness, which may limit daytime use but can be beneficial for pain-related sleep dysfunction.

Gabapentinoids, such as gabapentin and pregabalin, are centrally acting calcium channel blockers. This class of medication was initially developed for antiepileptic indications but has been extensively used, frequently off-label, in neuropathic pain conditions. Mechanism of action is thought to be primarily related to decreased activity in the ascending pain pathways by decreasing available glutamate and substance P, but they also appear to have some membrane stabilization activity. In patients with fibromyalgia, gabapentinoids are associated with improved pain, sleep, fatigue, and anxiety.[89] However, efficacy in chronic pelvic pain appears to be limited.[90] There is increasing concern about abuse or misuse of gabapentinoids, both with regard to nontherapeutic use and to risk for overdose when used concurrently with opioids.[91]

Cannabinoids are being increasingly used by patients with chronic pain conditions, despite fairly limited evidence regarding efficacy or safety. Cannabinoids are compounds derived from the cannabis plant. Over one hundred cannabinoids have been identified, but the 2 primary compounds are tetrahydrocannabinol (THC) and cannabidiol (CBD). THC is the cannabinoid associated with the classic psychoactive effects of cannabis, whereas CBD does not have psychoactive properties. Various cannabinoids have been studied in chronic pain conditions and demonstrate modest improvements in pain and sleep.[92,93] Side effects are variable but may include sedation, dry mouth, dry eye, nausea, and dizziness, and range from mild to moderate in most studies.[92,93] Despite limited data regarding efficacy, patients with chronic pain conditions are increasingly considering cannabinoids, particularly as more countries and localities have legalized medical and/or recreational use. More evidence-based data are needed regarding efficacy, dose, route, and safety considerations.

## Optimal Approach

The obvious question that arises after reviewing the aforementioned information is whether there is an algorithm or a validated stepwise approach that can be used when caring for patients with multiple chronic pain contributors. Everyone agrees that the trial-and-error approach is inefficient, inadequate, and demoralizing for patients and providers alike, but unfortunately, there is not yet a simple system that is able to effectively direct clinicians toward a personalized treatment plan for an individual patient.

The typical practice at our chronic pelvic pain and endometriosis referral clinic is to conduct a broad assessment for all potential pain contributors, including endometriosis, pelvic myofascial pain, COPCs, psychological conditions, and central sensitization at the initial consultation visit. We attempt to assess the degree to which each of these factors is driving pain symptoms, primarily based on an individual patient's history, symptoms, and physical examination. We discuss strategies to manage specific contributors, focusing on the fact that most patients require a multimodal, comprehensive approach. We are careful to present realistic expectations for anticipated responses to specific treatments and use shared decision making to decide how to proceed. When patients have a high degree of central sensitization, we preferentially recommend nonpharmacologic therapies, but admittedly access to cognitive behavior therapy and acupuncture is limited because of insurance coverage and provider availability in rural or underserved areas. When we feel that pharmacologic therapy is necessary, we attempt to individualize recommendations based on symptoms and historical responses to other medications. Because pelvic myofascial pain and sleep dysfunction are so prevalent among patients with chronic pelvic pain, we often begin with cyclobenzaprine or other muscle relaxants to target these symptoms in addition to shifting neurotransmitter activity. In a patient who has a mood disorder in addition to central sensitization, we may work with their primary care provider to initiate a trial of SNRI medication. An interdisciplinary approach is essential, as no single provider has adequate expertise to manage all these conditions alone. This comprehensive, multimodal, interdisciplinary approach has been described in the literature and was associated with significant improvement in pain and quality of life.[94]

## SUMMARY

Recognition of co-occurring COPCs can help clinicians provide better counseling and more tailored treatment recommendations for patients with chronic pelvic pain. Peripheral pain contributions should certainly be addressed using evidence-based management strategies, but clinicians must acknowledge the increased probability that pain may not improve sufficiently with peripheral treatments alone. Patients with co-occurring COPCs may benefit from the addition of treatments aimed at central sensitization, including pharmacologic and nonpharmacologic strategies.

## CLINICS CARE POINTS

- Evaluation of chronic pelvic pain should be comprehensive. Identification of one pain condition does not exclude the possibility of additional pain contributors.
- Consider pelvic myofascial pain and chronic overlapping pain conditions in your differential for patients with chronic pelvic pain.
- Empathetic communication and setting goals focused on functional improvements rather than pain resolution can improve patient satisfaction.
- Patients with multiple COPCs or central sensitization should have the opportunity to benefit from evidence-based peripheral treatments, such as medical or surgical treatment of endometriosis. But patients should be counseled that they are at higher risk for residual or recurrent pain, particularly when considering more invasive interventions such as surgery.
- Treating co-occurring psychological conditions can significantly improve the quality of life.
- Central sensitization is often present in patients with multiple COPCs. Multimodal management strategies that include nonpharmacologic and pharmacologic strategies can modify the impact of central sensitization and improve both pain and quality of life.

## DISCLOSURE

Dr S.R. Till is supported by NICHD 1K23HD09928301A1. Dr A. Schrepf is supported in part by NIH R43 DA046981. Dr S. As-Sanie is supported by NIH R01 HD088712. Dr S. As-Sanie is a consultant for Abbvie, Myovant, Bayer, and Eximis, and receives author royalties from UpToDate. The remaining authors have nothing to disclose.

## REFERENCES

1. Mathias SD, Kuppermann M, Liberman RF, et al. Chronic pelvic pain: prevalence, health-related quality of life, and economic correlates. Obstet Gynecol 1996; 87(3):321–7.
2. Zondervan KT, Yudkin PL, Vessey MP, et al. Chronic pelvic pain in the community–symptoms, investigations, and diagnoses. Am J Obstet Gynecol 2001; 184(6):1149–55.
3. Smith BH, Elliott AM, Hannaford PC, et al. Factors related to the onset and persistence of chronic back pain in the community: results from a general population follow-up study. Spine (Phila Pa 1976) 2004;29(9):1032–40.

4. Bergman S, Herrstrom P, Jacobsson LT, et al. Chronic widespread pain: a three year followup of pain distribution and risk factors. J Rheumatol 2002;29(4): 818–25.
5. Brummett CM, Urquhart AG, Hassett AL, et al. Characteristics of fibromyalgia independently predict poorer long-term analgesic outcomes following total knee and hip arthroplasty. Arthritis Rheumatol 2015;67(5):1386–94.
6. Schrepf A, Moser S, Harte SE, et al. Top down or bottom up? An observational investigation of improvement in fibromyalgia symptoms following hip and knee replacement. Rheumatology (Oxford) 2020;59(3):594–602.
7. Janda AM, As-Sanie S, Rajala B, et al. Fibromyalgia survey criteria are associated with increased postoperative opioid consumption in women undergoing hysterectomy. Anesthesiology 2015;122(5):1103–11.
8. Falcone T, Lebovic DI. Clinical management of endometriosis. Obstet Gynecol 2011;118(3):691–705.
9. Carter JE. Combined hysteroscopic and laparoscopic findings in patients with chronic pelvic pain. J Am Assoc Gynecol Laparosc 1994;2(1):43–7.
10. Balasch J, Creus M, Fabregues F, et al. Visible and non-visible endometriosis at laparoscopy in fertile and infertile women and in patients with chronic pelvic pain: a prospective study. Hum Reprod 1996;11(2):387–91.
11. D'Hooghe TM, Debrock S, Hill JA, et al. Endometriosis and subfertility: is the relationship resolved? Semin Reprod Med 2003;21(2):243–54.
12. Vercellini P, Trespidi L, De Giorgi O, et al. Endometriosis and pelvic pain: relation to disease stage and localization. Fertil Steril 1996;65(2):299–304.
13. Vercellini P, Fedele L, Aimi G, et al. Association between endometriosis stage, lesion type, patient characteristics and severity of pelvic pain symptoms: a multivariate analysis of over 1000 patients. Hum Reprod 2007;22(1):266–71.
14. Schrepf A, Phan V, Clemens JQ, et al. ICD-10 codes for the study of chronic overlapping pain conditions in administrative databases. J Pain 2020;21(1–2):59–70.
15. Bornstein J, Goldstein AT, Stockdale CK, et al. 2015 ISSVD, ISSWSH, and IPPS consensus terminology and classification of persistent vulvar pain and Vulvodynia. J Sex Med 2016;13(4):607–12.
16. Reed BD, Haefner HK, Harlow SD, et al. Reliability and validity of self-reported symptoms for predicting vulvodynia. Obstet Gynecol 2006;108(4):906–13.
17. Hanno PM, Erickson D, Moldwin R, et al. Diagnosis and treatment of interstitial cystitis/bladder pain syndrome: AUA guideline amendment. J Urol 2015;193(5): 1545–53.
18. Beissner F, Preibisch C, Schweizer-Arau A, et al. Psychotherapy with somatosensory stimulation for endometriosis-associated pain: the role of the anterior hippocampus. Biol Psychiatry 2017;84(10):734–42.
19. Berry SH, Elliott MN, Suttorp M, et al. Prevalence of symptoms of bladder pain syndrome/interstitial cystitis among adult females in the United States. J Urol 2011;186(2):540–4.
20. Longstreth GF, Thompson WG, Chey WD, et al. Functional bowel disorders. Gastroenterology 2006;130(5):1480–91.
21. Hungin AP, Whorwell PJ, Tack J, et al. The prevalence, patterns and impact of irritable bowel syndrome: an international survey of 40,000 subjects. Aliment Pharmacol Ther 2003;17(5):643–50.
22. Headache Classification Committee of the International Headache Society (IHS) The International Classification of Headache Disorders, 3rd edition. Cephalalgia 2018;38(1):1–211.

23. Russell MB, Levi N, Saltyte-Benth J, et al. Tension-type headache in adolescents and adults: a population based study of 33,764 twins. Eur J Epidemiol 2006; 21(2):153–60.
24. Greene CS. Managing the care of patients with temporomandibular disorders: a new guideline for care. J Am Dent Assoc 2010;141(9):1086–8.
25. Lipton JA, Ship JA, Larach-Robinson D. Estimated prevalence and distribution of reported orofacial pain in the United States. J Am Dent Assoc 1993;124(10): 115–21.
26. Johannes CB, Le TK, Zhou X, et al. The prevalence of chronic pain in United States adults: results of an Internet-based survey. J Pain 2010;11(11):1230–9.
27. Clauw DJ. Fibromyalgia: a clinical review. JAMA 2014;311(15):1547–55.
28. Wolfe F, Clauw DJ, Fitzcharles MA, et al. 2016 Revisions to the 2010/2011 fibromyalgia diagnostic criteria. Semin Arthritis Rheum 2016;46(3):319–29.
29. Ambrose K, Lyden AK, Clauw DJ. Applying exercise to the management of fibromyalgia. Curr Pain Headache Rep 2003;7(5):348–54.
30. Cleare AJ, Reid S, Chalder T, et al. Chronic fatigue syndrome. BMJ Clin Evid 2015;2015:1101.
31. Bates DW, Schmitt W, Buchwald D, et al. Prevalence of fatigue and chronic fatigue syndrome in a primary care practice. Arch Intern Med 1993;153(24): 2759–65.
32. Buchwald D, Umali P, Umali J, et al. Chronic fatigue and the chronic fatigue syndrome: prevalence in a Pacific Northwest health care system. Ann Intern Med 1995;123(2):81–8.
33. Mills SEE, Nicolson KP, Smith BH. Chronic pain: a review of its epidemiology and associated factors in population-based studies. Br J Anaesth 2019;123(2): e273–83.
34. van Hecke O, Torrance N, Smith BH. Chronic pain epidemiology and its clinical relevance. Br J Anaesth 2013;111(1):13–8.
35. Warren JW, Langenberg P, Clauw DJ. The number of existing functional somatic syndromes (FSSs) is an important risk factor for new, different FSSs. J Psychosom Res 2013;74(1):12–7.
36. Rahmioglu N, Nyholt DR, Morris AP, et al. Genetic variants underlying risk of endometriosis: insights from meta-analysis of eight genome-wide association and replication datasets. Hum Reprod Update 2014;20(5):702–16.
37. Kato K, Sullivan PF, Evengard B, et al. A population-based twin study of functional somatic syndromes. Psychol Med 2009;39(3):497–505.
38. Laurell K, Larsson B, Eeg-Olofsson O. Headache in schoolchildren: association with other pain, family history and psychosocial factors. Pain 2005;119(1–3): 150–8.
39. Allen-Brady K, Norton P, Cannon-Albright L. Risk of associated conditions in relatives of subjects with interstial cystitis. Female Pelvic Med Reconstr Surg 2015; 21(2):93.
40. Harte SE, Harris RE, Clauw DJ. The neurobiology of central sensitization. J Appl Biobehav Res 2018;23(2):e12137.
41. Harte SE, Schrepf A, Gallop R, et al. Quantitative assessment of nonpelvic pressure pain sensitivity in urologic chronic pelvic pain syndrome: a MAPP Research Network study. Pain 2019;160(6):1270–80.
42. As-Sanie S, Kim J, Schmidt-Wilcke T, et al. Functional connectivity is associated with altered brain chemistry in women with endometriosis-associated chronic pelvic pain. J Pain 2016;17(1):1–13.

43. Petzke F, Clauw DJ, Ambrose K, et al. Increased pain sensitivity in fibromyalgia: effects of stimulus type and mode of presentation. Pain 2003;105(3):403–13.
44. Palacios-Ceña M, Lima Florencio L, Natália Ferracini G, et al. Women with chronic and episodic migraine exhibit similar widespread pressure pain sensitivity. Pain Med 2016;17(11):2127–33.
45. Stabell N, Stubhaug A, Flægstad T, et al. Increased pain sensitivity among adults reporting irritable bowel syndrome symptoms in a large population-based study. Pain 2013;154(3):385–92.
46. Winger A, Kvarstein G, Wyller VB, et al. Pain and pressure pain thresholds in ad-olescents with chronic fatigue syndrome and healthy controls: a cross-sectional study. BMJ Open 2014;4(10):e005920.
47. Nimnuan C, Rabe-Hesketh S, Wessely S, et al. How many functional somatic syn-dromes? J Psychosom Res 2001;51(4):549–57.
48. Schrepf A, Williams DA, Gallop R, et al. Sensory sensitivity and symptom severity represent unique dimensions of chronic pain: a MAPP Research Network study. Pain 2018;159(10):2002–11.
49. Grace PM, Tawfik VL, Svensson CI, et al. The neuroimmunology of chronic pain: from rodents to humans. J Neurosci 2020;41(5):855–65.
50. Schrepf A, Bradley CS, O'Donnell M, et al. Toll-like receptor 4 and comorbid pain in Interstitial Cystitis/Bladder Pain Syndrome: a multidisciplinary approach to the study of chronic pelvic pain research network study. Brain Behav Immun 2015;49: 66–74.
51. Schrepf A, O'Donnell M, Luo Y, et al. Inflammation and inflammatory control in interstitial cystitis/bladder pain syndrome: associations with painful symptoms. Pain 2014;155:1755–61.
52. Evans SF, Kwok YH, Solterbeck A, et al. Toll-like receptor responsiveness of pe-ripheral blood mononuclear cells in young women with dysmenorrhea. J Pain Res 2020;13:503–16.
53. Mckernan DP, Gaszner G, Quigley EM, et al. Altered peripheral toll-like receptor responses in the irritable bowel syndrome. Aliment Pharmacol Ther 2011;33(9): 1045–52.
54. Fitzgerald CM, Neville CE, Mallinson T, et al. Pelvic floor muscle examination in female chronic pelvic pain. J Reprod Med 2011;56(3–4):117–22.
55. Sedighimehr N, Manshadi FD, Shokouhi N, et al. Pelvic musculoskeletal dysfunc-tions in women with and without chronic pelvic pain. J Bodyw Mov Ther 2018; 22(1):92–6.
56. Williams DA, Schilling S. Advances in the assessment of fibromyalgia. Rheum Dis Clin North Am 2009;35(2):339–57.
57. Falcone T, Flyckt R. Clinical management of endometriosis. Obstet Gynecol 2018; 131(3):557–71.
58. Rosen NO, Dawson SJ, Brooks M, et al. Treatment of vulvodynia: pharmacolog-ical and non-pharmacological approaches. Drugs 2019;79(5):483–93.
59. Vandyken C, Hilton S. Physical therapy in the treatment of central pain mecha-nisms for female sexual pain. Sex Med Rev 2017;5(1):20–30.
60. Bryant C, Cockburn R, Plante A-F, et al. The psychological profile of women pre-senting to a multidisciplinary clinic for chronic pelvic pain: high levels of psycho-logical dysfunction and implications for practice. J Pain Res 2016;9:1049–56.
61. Miller-Matero LR, Saulino C, Clark S, et al. When treating the pain is not enough: a multidisciplinary approach for chronic pelvic pain. Arch Womens Ment Health 2016;19(2):349–54.

62. Romão APMS, Gorayeb R, Romão GS, et al. High levels of anxiety and depression have a negative effect on quality of life of women with chronic pelvic pain. Int J Clin Pract 2009;63(5):707–11.
63. Lorençatto C, Petta CA, Navarro MJ, et al. Depression in women with endometriosis with and without chronic pelvic pain. Acta Obstet Gynecol Scand 2006; 85(1):88–92.
64. Williams DA. The importance of psychological assessment in chronic pain. Curr Opin Urol 2013;23(6):554–9.
65. Yosef A, Allaire C, Williams C, et al. Multifactorial contributors to the severity of chronic pelvic pain in women. Am J Obstet Gynecol 2016;215(6):760.e1–14.
66. Till SR, As-Sanie S, Schrepf A. Psychology of chronic pelvic pain: prevalence, neurobiological vulnerabilities, and treatment. Clin Obstet Gynecol 2019;62(1): 22–36.
67. de Heer EW, Ten Have M, van Marwijk HWJ, et al. Pain as a risk factor for common mental disorders. Results from the Netherlands Mental Health Survey and Incidence Study-2: a longitudinal, population-based study. Pain 2018;159(4): 712–8.
68. Hilderink PH, Burger H, Deeg DJ, et al. The temporal relation between pain and depression: results from the longitudinal aging study Amsterdam. Psychosom Med 2012;74(9):945–51.
69. Cella D, Riley W, Stone A, et al. The Patient-Reported Outcomes Measurement Information System (PROMIS) developed and tested its first wave of adult self-reported health outcome item banks: 2005–2008. J Clin Epidemiol 2010;63(11): 1179–94.
70. Wolfe F, Clauw DJ, Fitzcharles M-A, et al. Fibromyalgia criteria and severity scales for clinical and epidemiological studies: a modification of the ACR Preliminary Diagnostic Criteria for Fibromyalgia. J Rheumatol 2011;38(6):1113–22.
71. Neville SJ, Clauw AD, Moser SE, et al. Association between the 2011 fibromyalgia survey criteria and multisite pain sensitivity in knee osteoarthritis. Clin J Pain 2018;34(10):909–17.
72. Gonçalves AV, Barros NF, Bahamondes L. The practice of hatha yoga for the treatment of pain associated with endometriosis. J Altern Complement Med 2017;23(1):45–52.
73. Johannesson E, Simrén M, Strid H, et al. Physical activity improves symptoms in irritable bowel syndrome: a randomized controlled trial. Am J Gastroenterol 2011; 106(5):915–22.
74. Santiago MDS, Carvalho DdS, Gabbai AA, et al. Amitriptyline and aerobic exercise or amitriptyline alone in the treatment of chronic migraine: a randomized comparative study. Arq Neuropsiquiatr 2014;72(11):851–5.
75. Turner JA, Holtzman S, Mancl L. Mediators, moderators, and predictors of therapeutic change in cognitive-behavioral therapy for chronic pain. Pain 2007;127(3): 276–86.
76. Okifuji A, Ackerlind S. Behavioral medicine approaches to pain. Anesthesiol Clin 2007;25(4):709–19, v.
77. Lindström S, Kvist LJ. Treatment of Provoked Vulvodynia in a Swedish cohort using desensitization exercises and cognitive behavioral therapy. BMC Womens Health 2015;15:108.
78. Meissner K, Schweizer-Arau A, Limmer A, et al. Psychotherapy with somatosensory stimulation for endometriosis-associated pain. Obstet Gynecol 2016;128(5): 1134–42.

79. Ford AC, Talley NJ, Schoenfeld PS, et al. Efficacy of antidepressants and psychological therapies in irritable bowel syndrome: systematic review and meta-analysis. Gut 2009;58(3):367–78.
80. Lazaridou A, Kim J, Cahalan CM, et al. Effects of Cognitive-Behavioral Therapy (CBT) on brain connectivity supporting catastrophizing in fibromyalgia. Clin J Pain 2017;33(3):215–21.
81. Wayne PM, Kerr CE, Schnyer RN, et al. Japanese-style acupuncture for endometriosis-related pelvic pain in adolescents and young women: results of a randomized sham-controlled trial. J Pediatr Adolesc Gynecol 2008;21(5):247–57.
82. Rubi-Klein K, Kucera-Sliutz E, Nissel H, et al. Is acupuncture in addition to conventional medicine effective as pain treatment for endometriosis? A randomised controlled cross-over trial. Eur J Obstet Gynecol Reprod Biol 2010;153(1):90–3.
83. Xu Y, Zhao W, Li T, et al. Effects of acupuncture for the treatment of endometriosis-related pain: a systematic review and meta-analysis. PLoS One 2017;12(10):e0186616.
84. Arnold LM. Duloxetine and other antidepressants in the treatment of patients with fibromyalgia. Pain Med 2007;8(Suppl 2):S63–74.
85. Gendreau RM, Thorn MD, Gendreau JF, et al. Efficacy of milnacipran in patients with fibromyalgia. J Rheumatol 2005;32(10):1975–85.
86. Moore RA, Derry S, Aldington D, et al. Amitriptyline for neuropathic pain and fibromyalgia in adults. Cochrane Database Syst Rev 2012;12:CD008242.
87. Tofferi JK, Jackson JL, O'Malley PG. Treatment of fibromyalgia with cyclobenzaprine: a meta-analysis. Arthritis Rheum 2004;51(1):9–13.
88. Moldofsky H, Harris HW, Archambault WT, et al. Effects of bedtime very low dose cyclobenzaprine on symptoms and sleep physiology in patients with fibromyalgia syndrome: a double-blind randomized placebo-controlled study. J Rheumatol 2011;38(12):2653–63.
89. Häuser W, Bernardy K, Uçeyler N, et al. Treatment of fibromyalgia syndrome with gabapentin and pregabalin–a meta-analysis of randomized controlled trials. Pain 2009;145(1–2):69–81.
90. Horne AW, Vincent K, Hewitt CA, et al. Gabapentin for chronic pelvic pain in women (GaPP2): a multicentre, randomised, double-blind, placebo-controlled trial. Lancet 2020;396(10255):909–17.
91. Evoy KE, Sadrameli S, Contreras J, et al. Abuse and misuse of pregabalin and gabapentin: a systematic review update. Drugs 2021;81(1):125–56.
92. Lynch ME, Campbell F. Cannabinoids for treatment of chronic non-cancer pain; a systematic review of randomized trials. Br J Clin Pharmacol 2011;72(5):735–44.
93. Boehnke KF, Gagnier JJ, Matallana L, et al. Cannabidiol use for fibromyalgia: prevalence of use and perceptions of effectiveness in a large online survey. J Pain 2021;22(5):556–66.
94. Allaire C, Williams C, Bodmer-Roy S, et al. Chronic pelvic pain in an interdisciplinary setting: 1-year prospective cohort. Am J Obstet Gynecol 2018;218(1):114.e1–2.

# A Practical Approach to Fertility Considerations in Endometriosis Surgery

Jenna Gale, MSc, MD, FRCSC[a,b,c,d,*],
Sukhbir Sony Singh, MD, FRCSC[a,b,c]

## KEYWORDS

- Endometriosis • Minimally invasive surgery • Fertility • Deep endometriosis
- Endometriomas • In vitro fertilization

## KEY POINTS

- Endometriosis affects 5% to 10% of reproductive-age women, and the prevalence among women with infertility has been reported as high as 50%.
- Endometriosis surgery can improve the chance of spontaneous conception; however, surgery for endometriosis-related infertility requires thoughtful evaluation, planning, and patient counseling.
- In the absence of other surgical indications (ie, pain), there is a lack of good quality evidence to support first-line surgery to improve fertility treatment outcomes.
- A personalized approach to each patient should consider symptoms including pelvic pain, past fertility and surgical interventions, extent of disease, and the need to treat coexisting conditions.

## INTRODUCTION

Endometriosis is a disease characterized by the presence of endometrium-like epithelium and/or stroma outside the endometrium and myometrium, usually with an associated inflammatory process.[1] It is a common condition among reproductive-age individuals assigned female sex at birth and is often associated with infertility. Approximately 1 in 10 girls and women, and unmeasured numbers of transgender, nonbinary, and gender diverse individuals, will have endometriosis. Among women with pelvic pain, the prevalence of endometriosis increases to 50% to 70%.[2] The prevalence

[a] Department of Obstetrics, Gynecology and Newborn Care, The Ottawa Hospital, 501 Smyth Road, Ottawa, Ontario K1H 8L6, Canada; [b] Faculty of Medicine, University of Ottawa, Roger Guindon Hall, 451 Smyth Road, Ottawa, Ontario K1H 8M5, Canada; [c] Ottawa Hospital Research Institute, 1053 Carling Avenue, Ottawa, Ontario, K1Y 4E9, Canada; [d] Ottawa Fertility Centre, 955 Green Valley Crescent, Ottawa, Ontario, K2C 3V4, Canada
* Corresponding author. Ottawa Fertility Centre, 955 Green Valley Crescent, Ottawa, Ontario, K2C 3V4, Canada.
E-mail address: jgale@toh.ca
Twitter: @DrJennaGale (J.G.)

Obstet Gynecol Clin N Am 49 (2022) 241–256
https://doi.org/10.1016/j.ogc.2022.02.007
0889-8545/22/Crown Copyright © 2022 Published by Elsevier Inc. All rights reserved.

among patients with infertility has been reported as high as 50%, and infertile patients are 6 to 8 times more likely to have endometriosis than fertile women.[2,3]

The mechanism by which endometriosis impacts fertility is likely multi-factorial and may involve the entire reproductive tract through structural and functional impairment. Severe adhesive disease associated with advanced endometriosis is an obvious impairment to fertility, affecting ovum release and capture; however, the full extent of the association of endometriosis with infertility remains unresolved. Endometriosis has been implicated at many levels beyond distorted pelvic anatomy, including cycle irregularity, impairment of follicular growth, lower oocyte and embryo quality, luteal phase dysfunction, altered peritoneal function, impaired fertilization, and reduced implantation rates, among others.[4,5] Although the relationship between endometriosis and infertility is indisputable, accurately predicting fertility among those with endometriosis is challenging.

Endometriosis has several different phenotypes (peritoneal, ovarian endometriomas, and deep disease) and may also be associated with other pathologies such as adenomyosis and uterine fibroids. The lack of accounting for coexisting conditions can lead to diagnostic biases when evaluating fertility outcomes among patients with endometriosis. As a result of these challenges, predicting which patient will benefit from surgery, from both a quality of life (QOL) and fertility perspective, is difficult. In this article, we will discuss important considerations with regards to fertility and endometriosis surgery, including an approach to selecting the appropriate candidate for surgery, surgical techniques, and special considerations.

### Endometriosis Staging

The American Society for Reproductive Medicine (ASRM) scoring system is the most widely used classification system. It categorizes endometriosis into 4 stages of minimal (stage I), mild (stage II), moderate (stage III), and severe (stage IV)[6] (**Fig. 1**). The ASRM classification system, however, does not correlate with symptoms or prognosis of endometriosis, and heterogeneity of symptoms is high among patients with endometriosis.[2] The ASRM scoring also does not accurately reflect deep endometriosis (DE) involvement which limits its use in those cases.

While many other classification systems have been proposed, a recent systematic review on endometriosis staging systems concluded that there is a lack of agreement on classification globally and "no or very little correlation with patient outcomes."[7] A new surgical complexity classification system proposed by the AAGL helps to provide a practical approach to predicting/describing surgical complexity better than the ASRM staging previously proposed.[8]

The classification systems discussed above, however, have limited utility in predicting pregnancy outcomes after gynecologic surgery for endometriosis. The endometriosis fertility index (EFI) is a clinical tool developed to predict postoperative spontaneous pregnancy rates among patients after surgical diagnosis and treatment of endometriosis[9] (**Fig. 2**). The tool was developed to provide reassurance for patients with good prognosis for spontaneous conception, and triaging those with poor prognosis to assisted reproductive technology (ART) and avoid wasted time. This tool has been shown to have good inter-expert clinical agreement[10] and has demonstrated good predictive performance in a recent systematic review and meta-analysis.[11]

---

**Clinical tip**

The use of endometriosis staging systems helps document surgical findings, which may improve communication among care providers. The EFI may help guide postoperative fertility management decisions.

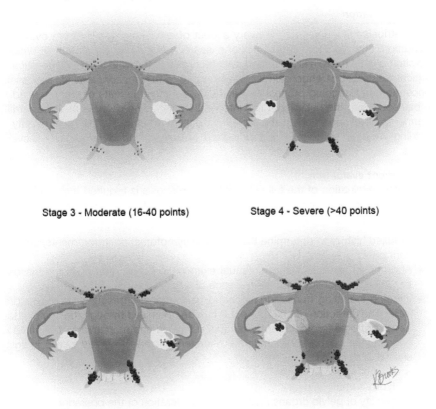

**Fig. 1.** American Society for Reproductive Medicine (ASRM) endometriosis scoring system. (*Adapted from* Revised American Society for Reproductive Medicine classification of endometriosis: 1996. Fertil Steril. 1997;67(5):817-821. https://doi.org/10.1016/s0015-0282(97)81391-x; with permission. Reprinted by permission from the American Society for Reproductive Medicine.)

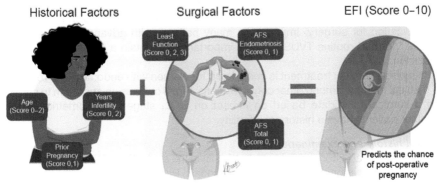

*American Fertility Society (AFS) now the American Society for Reproductive Medicine (ASRM)

**Fig. 2.** Endometriosis fertility index (EFI). (*Adapted from* Revised American Society for Reproductive Medicine classification of endometriosis: 1996. Fertil Steril. 1997;67(5):817-821. https://doi.org/10.1016/s0015-0282(97)81391-x; with permission. Reprinted by permission from the American Society for Reproductive Medicine.)

## Clinical Evaluation

Endometriosis influences almost every aspect of a patients' fertility from ovulation, fertilization, embryo implantation, risk of miscarriage, and risk in pregnancy. What is less clear is what the role is for surgery with regards to improving fertility. Theoretically, surgical treatment of endometriosis might improve the environment for successful conception and ongoing pregnancy. However, potential benefits of surgery need to be balanced with the risk of surgical intervention, including delay in assisted fertility treatments. The approach to the individual patient whereby fertility is a priority in deciding whether surgery is recommended is unique and dependent on several factors.

### Initial patient evaluation

A complete evaluation of the full extent of endometriosis is required through history, physical examination, and imaging.[12] A thorough initial work-up is imperative and should include:

- Detailed history to determine the extent of symptoms, past treatments, and patient goals;
- Abdominal, speculum and bimanual examination to evaluate ovarian masses, pelvic organ mobility and the presence of DE;
- Imaging including transabdominal and transvaginal ultrasound (TVUS) (and/or MRI). The detection of endometriosis can be optimized through the use of a targeted protocol for sonographer-acquired images and maneuvers at the time of endovaginal sonographic imaging.[13] Systematic and targeted pelvic imaging should evaluate for signs of:
  - Ovarian endometriomas
  - Hydro/hematosalpinx
  - Mobility of pelvic organs (sliding sign), obliteration of the posterior cul-de-sac
  - DE deposits, with or without bowel involvement
  - Hydro-ureter, hydronephrosis
- Full evaluation of the risk of malignancy, with the risk of malignancy scoring when applicable

After a thorough clinical evaluation of the extent of endometriosis and its impact on QOL and an individual patients' current or future desire for pregnancy, a tailored approach should be taken regarding whether to proceed with surgery. In particular, adequate pelvic imaging to understand the full extent of endometriosis can help inform the indication for surgery. Importantly, many patients with advanced disease may have a "normal" routine TVUS and it is important to maintain a high level of clinical suspicion.

In general, surgical treatment is considered for women with endometriosis resistant to medical therapy, among other considerations. **Fig. 3** outlines an approach to selecting a surgical candidate based on impact on QOL, stage of endometriosis, and whether patients have a history of infertility.

### Clinical history and examination

A detailed clinical history is imperative to assist in the evaluation of the extent of endometriosis and its impact on patient QOL and goals. Particular attention should be paid to symptoms that could be attributed to endometriosis. Specifically, the following details should be sought on history[12]:

- Age;
- Body mass index (BMI);

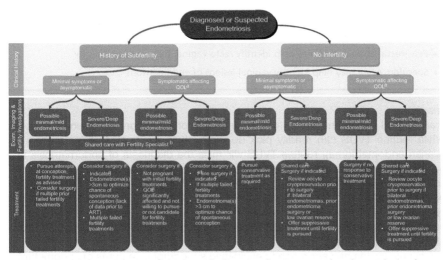

**Fig. 3.** Approach to managing patients with diagnosed or suspected endometriosis who are contemplating fertility. <sup>a</sup>QOL, quality of life. <sup>b</sup>Shared care with a fertility specialist where available. <sup>c</sup>Indications: rule out malignancy, manage visceral obstruction and/or patient request.

- Number and outcome of prior pregnancies;
- Subfertility and its duration;
- Outcome of fertility consultation and investigations;
- Prior fertility treatment(s) and their outcome(s);
- Current fertility goals (ie, actively trying for pregnancy, long-term fertility preservation, undecided)
- Menstrual history;
- Prior gynecologic surgery (including surgery for endometriosis);
- Pain (pain with menses, intercourse, urination, bowel movements, chronic pelvic pain);
- Blood in the urine or stool;
- Results of prior pelvic imaging.

The pain should be further explored, with quantification on a scale of 0 to 10 or with the use of a visual analog scale (VAS).

A thorough examination, as described by Vilasagar and colleagues,[12] for those with suspected endometriosis and/or pelvic pain with infertility is crucial. Identifying obvious cul-de-sac nodularity, pelvic masses, and areas of pain will guide next steps and imaging.

---

**Key Examination Tips**

- An abdominal and pelvic exam should assess for sites of pain and identify:
  - Masses
  - Allodynia or hyperalgesia
  - Muscle tone and tenderness (pelvic floor and abdominal wall)
  - Previous scars or injury
  - Nodularity along the vaginal fornices or cul-de-sac

○ Uterine mobility and axis
○ Neurological patterns of pain or sensory deficits
• Pelvi-rectal examination may help identify recto-vaginal fullness or nodularity
• Speculum exam may help identify vaginal lesions of endometriosis

## Imaging

Transvaginal ultrasound is the first-line imaging for the diagnosis of endometriosis. While routine TVUS can readily pick up more obvious signs of endometriosis (ie, ovarian endometrioma), routine TVUS will miss the diagnosis of endometriosis in 3 out of 4 patients who have this prevalent condition.[14] Therefore, routine pelvic ultrasound is a valuable first-line imaging; however, patients with a higher degree of suspicion of endometriosis (based on the history of physical examination described above), or all patients with the history of infertility given the prevalence of endometriosis among this population, should undergo more detailed systematic imaging evaluation for endometriosis.

A simple systematic approach to evaluating sonographic features of endometriosis was developed and validated to improve the diagnostic accuracy of TVUS and standardize nomenclature.[15] This systematic approach to TVUS evaluates "soft markers" (ie, site-specific tenderness and ovarian mobility), "sliding sign" (suggestion of posterior cul-de-sac adhesion involvement) and assesses for DE nodules.[15] Additionally, pelvic imaging should comment on signs of hydro-hematosalpinx, hydroureter/hydronephrosis. MRI may assist in further preoperative mapping of endometriosis, especially in cases of multi-organ involvement especially beyond the pelvis and in cases whereby there is a lack of access to expert-guided ultrasound.[16] A standardized approach for MRI and ultrasound are essential for proper communication with surgeons and care teams.[16]

## Preparing for Surgery

A multidisciplinary approach to the patient undergoing surgery whereby fertility is a priority is imperative. Patients should undergo preoperative referral to a fertility specialist for fertility investigations and counseling of their options to make a fully informed decision regarding their care.

Preoperative focused fertility investigations include:

• Ultrasound to evaluate ovarian accessibility for oocyte retrieval
• Partner semen analysis (when indicated)
• Ovarian reserve testing including anti-Mullerian hormone (AMH) level and antral follicle count
• Tubal patency evaluated through hysterosalpingogram (HSG) or hysterosalpingo-contrast sonography (HyCoSy)

## Clinical tip

Tubal patency evaluation is important preoperatively for surgical planning. In cases of hydrosalpinx that communicate with the uterine cavity (patent cornua), salpingectomy should be undertaken before ART treatment. Communicating hydrosalpinges are associated with lower implantation rates at the time of embryo transfer,[17] and fimbrioplasty is of limited utility. In cases of bilateral salpingectomy, patients must be fully informed that this will preclude spontaneous conception, given that although the chance of spontaneous pregnancy is rare with bilateral hydrosalpinges/blocked tubes, patients not wishing to undergo or not candidates for ART may opt against surgery.

Among cases of suspected tubal blockage without hydrosalpinx, the decision for salpingectomy is individualized and factors that influence this decision include age, whether they are a candidate for ART, willingness to undergo ART, history of prior ectopic pregnancies, and the appearance and patency of the fallopian at the time of surgery.

### Preoperative fertility preservation

In any case of suspected or diagnosed endometriosis, presurgical discussion of fertility preservation (either through oocyte or embryo cryopreservation) should be considered, secondary to the potential negative impact of the surgery on ovarian reserve and ovarian accessibility for a future oocyte retrieval procedure.

There is a paucity of evidence surrounding the role of fertility preservation for patients with endometriosis before surgery. As a result of lack of data on the survival rate of cryopreserve oocytes, reproductive potential, patient satisfaction, and cost-effectiveness, oocyte cryopreservation is not standard practice befpre surgery for advanced endometriosis. However, there may be a role for preoperative fertility preservation in specific circumstances, particularly when the risk of damage to ovarian reserve or premature ovarian insufficiency is high. Patients with (1) bilateral endometriomas, (2) prior excision of unilateral endometriomas who require surgery for contralateral recurrence[18], and (3) low ovarian reserve may benefit from preoperative fertility preservation. However, fertility preservation among patients with low ovarian reserve or endometrioma(s) is not always feasible or possible.

### Clinical tip

Consider referral to a fertility specialist for counseling about the option of fertility preservation before surgery for endometriosis for patients with bilateral ovarian endometriomas, prior excision of ovarian endometriomas, and/or low ovarian reserve.

### Preoperative counseling

In addition to preoperative counseling regarding the option of fertility preservation, risks and benefits of laparoscopic treatment of endometriosis must be reviewed. Unfortunately, due to the significant heterogeneity in surgical approaches, disease variation, and patient comorbid factors, there is no simple overall risk "number" that can be quoted. Each case is unique and requires an individual discussion including the following risks:

- Risk of reduction in ovarian reserve (and lower postoperative oocyte yield for ART);
- Risk of oophorectomy or premature ovarian insufficiency;
- Risk of ovarian inaccessibility for future oocyte retrieval and;
- Risk of postoperative adhesions causing tubal dysfunction or blockage.

### Surgical Indications for Endometriosis-Related Subfertility

### Minimal and mild endometriosis

Laparoscopic treatment of minimal or mild endometriosis is associated with a small but significant improvement in live birth rates.[19,20] Two randomized controlled trials (RCTs) have studied whether laparoscopic treatment of endometriosis, by ablation or excision, is associated with improved spontaneous pregnancy rates. The first study, which included 341 infertile women ages 20 to 39, found that women randomized to the treatment group were almost twice as likely to achieve pregnancy over a 36-month follow-up period (with an increased monthly pregnancy rate from 3% to 6%).[19] In contrast to this study, a second RCT of 101 patients did not show a difference in pregnancy rates.[20] When the results of these 2 studies are combined, the number needed to treat (NNT) to achieve one additional pregnancy among women with mild or moderate endometriosis is 12.[5] However, the challenge in interpreting this data is that not all patients with infertility who undergo diagnostic laparoscopy for possible endometriosis will have minimal or mild endometriosis, and therefore if we consider a conservative common prevalence of 30% among women with unexplained infertility, the adjusted NNT would be 40.[5] As a result of these findings, international guidelines do not support the use of routine diagnostic laparoscopy for couples with unexplained infertility to rule out and potentially treatment minimal to mild endometriosis.

Among patients with known or suspected endometriosis, surgery may be reviewed as an option in the setting of failed treatment with superovulation with intrauterine insemination (SO-IUI) or ovulation induction, before IVF. Treatment with SO-IUI is not generally recommended for patients with more advanced endometriosis (given distorted pelvic anatomy and altered tubal function). However, there is a lack of evidence to suggest that failed SO-IUI treatment is an indication for surgical treatment of endometriosis, and given that IVF maximizes cycle fecundity among patients with endometriosis,[5] IVF is generally the next step among patients who fail SO-IUI treatment. The counseling around the potential risks and benefits of surgery for these patients is similar to those with infertility who have not attempted IVF.

### Clinical tip

Indications for surgery among patients with unexplained infertility and suspected minimal to mild endometriosis (ASRM Stage 1–2) include:

- Endometriosis-related symptoms with a goal to improve QOL.
- When fertility treatment options are not accessible (ie, due to cost or geography) or the patient is not a candidate for or declines fertility interventions.

### Ovarian Endometriomas

Approximately 17% to 44% of patients with endometriosis have ovarian endometriomas.[21] More easily appreciated on diagnostic evaluation through TVUS, ovarian endometriomas are a marker for more extensive pelvic and intestinal disease, as only approximately 1% of patients with endometriomas have ovarian disease exclusively.[22] Additionally, among patients with ovarian endometriomas, deep lesions are more severe with an increased rate of vaginal, intestinal and ureteral involvement.[23]

Laparoscopic cystectomy for ovarian endometriomas greater than 3 cm is associated with improved fertility relative to cyst drainage and coagulation.[24] For patients who are subsequently attempting to conceive after surgical management of endometrioma, excision is associated with an increased spontaneous pregnancy rate among patients who had documented prior subfertility (OR 5.21, CI 2.04–13.29).[25] In addition to the size of the endometriomas, indications for surgery include inability to access follicles as a result of the endometrioma(s) among patients who will undergo ART, rapid growth and suspicious features noted on ultrasound.[18,26]

Current evidence does not suggest that cystectomy improves fertility outcomes among patients before IVF.[27] Outcomes after IVF including implantation rates, clinical pregnancy rates and live birth rates are similar when comparing patients who undergo cystectomy for endometrioma versus controls.[28] Ovarian endometrioma cystectomy is not routinely recommended before IVF and is most often considered before IVF for patients whereby access to follicles is impaired, who have significant pain and/or atypical imaging findings requiring pathologic diagnosis.[5]

Patients with endometriomas (without surgery) have lower ovarian reserve and a steeper decline in ovarian reserve.[29] Additionally, patients who undergo ovarian cystectomy for endometriomas have a reduction in the ovarian reserve as measured by AMH level.[30] These AMH levels may recover over time; however, the rate and degree of recovery of AMH varies. Nonfavorable factors that are associated with impaired recovery include baseline infertility and increased cyst burden.[30] Patients with larger endometriomas or bilateral endometriomas are at increased risk of further diminished ovarian reserve after ovarian cystectomy. The risk of postsurgical premature ovarian insufficiency after excision of bilateral endometriomas is approximately 2% to 3%.[31]

Recurrence of endometriomas is a significant concern, and the recurrence of endometriomas may be as high as 50% without suppressive therapy.[32,33] Younger age at surgery, stage of endometriosis, size of the endometrioma and previous medical or surgical treatment are suggested risk factors for endometrioma recurrence.[32] Although a barrier to conception, the use of medical therapy is effective at reducing the risk of recurrence.[33,34] Therefore, the pursuit of ART is typically recommended among patients trying to conceive if conception has not occurred in a relatively short time period after surgery.

### Clinical tip: for ovarian endometriomas

- Consider surgery for the patient with infertility if endometrioma size greater than 3 cm and there is a desire for *spontaneous conception.*
- Consider surgery if there are rapid growth or suspicious features of the endometrioma on ultrasound, the inability to access ovarian follicles for oocyte retrieval, and/or symptoms significantly impacting the QOL.
- Surgery should be cautiously used in cases of ovarian endometriomas due to the risk of reduction in ovarian reserve or premature ovarian insufficiency.
- Repeat or bilateral ovarian surgery further increases the risk of damage to ovarian reserve.
- Postoperative recurrence of endometriomas is high without medical suppression.

### Deep Endometriosis

Deep endometriosis (DE) is defined as endometrium-like tissue lesions extending on or under the peritoneal surface. They are usually nodular, able to invade adjacent structures, and associated with fibrosis and disruption of normal anatomy. The predominant symptom of DE is pain. The type of painful symptoms and the intensity of pain are related to the anatomic location and the depth of penetration of the DE lesions, respectively.[35]

Studies evaluating fertility outcomes after surgery for DE are heterogeneous and inherently biased. Among patients who pursue surgery for DE, the spontaneous pregnancy rate after surgical resection of DE is 21% to 49%.[36] There are no RCTs evaluating whether first-line IVF versus first-line surgery for infertile patients with DE yields better live birth rates. In a recent meta-analysis of 12 cohort studies, none of which were RCTs, studies were consistent in demonstrating a benefit for surgery before IVF.[37] These results need to be evaluated with extreme caution, given the high heterogeneity in the reported data and the significant risk of selection and allocation bias. As an example, most fertility specialists would not recommend surgery for those who have a low ovarian reserve before IVF. These patients will have inherently lower success rates with IVF, thus significantly biasing nonrandomized study results.

Randomized control trials are necessary to determine whether surgery before IVF among patients with DE leads to higher live birth rates. There is insufficient evidence to routinely recommend surgery before IVF for patients with DE. Currently, the main indications for surgical management of DE-related infertility are to manage pain or visceral (bowel, ureteric) obstruction. For patients with the recurrence of DE after a first surgical excision in experienced hands, among whom fertility is the main goal of treatment, repeated excision is not recommended.[38,39] Among these patients, ART leads to better results compared with a repeat operation.

Bowel endometriosis presents a particular challenge for the gynecologic surgeon and fertility specialist. A skilled, experienced multidisciplinary team comfortable with bowel endometriosis is a necessity for optimal outcomes and low complication rates. However, there is no clear consensus on whether surgery before ART or direct to ART is preferred for patients with DE and bowel involvement.[40] Additionally, although surgical management of bowel endometriosis is associated with significant improvement in overall well-being, it presents significant intra and postoperative risk including, but not limited to, rectovaginal fistula formation, hemorrhage, infections, conversion to laparotomy, bladder and bowel dysfunction.[40] Complications after bowel surgery for endometriosis, even in expert centers, are reported between 10% and 25%, which should be discussed in advance with the patient and their family.[41] It is generally accepted that for asymptomatic patients with bowel endometriosis whereby fertility is the primary goal, ART is the first-line option.[40]

The role of surgery among patients with multiple prior failed ART cycles/embryo transfers is not clear. One study evaluated surgery after repeated IVF failures and found that after surgical treatment, 42% of patients delivered (9% spontaneous conceptions and the remainder through additional IVF).[42] The study setting was highly unique environment of multiple funded IVF cycles, whereby the average number of cycles was 6 and for many of these patients this was not their first surgery for endometriosis; therefore, this data is difficult to extrapolate to other populations. However, there is likely a role of surgery among patients with repeated IVF failures before further fertility treatment.

### Clinical tip: surgery for deep endometriosis

- The management of bowel endometriosis requires careful consideration of symptoms, patient goals, and an experienced team with surgical and fertility experience.
- Approximately one-third of patients who have surgery for DE, in centers with expertise, will achieve spontaneous conception.
- ART is generally chosen as first line over surgery for patients wishing to conceive, whereby fertility is the primary concern.
- There is likely a role for surgery among patients with repeated failed ART cycles.

### Mitigation of Risk in Pregnancy

Patients with endometriosis are possibly at increased risk of pregnancy complications, including placenta previa, preterm birth, low birth weight, and cesarean delivery, among other pregnancy complications, compared with patients without endometriosis.[43] It is unknown whether surgical treatment of endometriosis before pregnancy will reduce these possible associated risks in future pregnancy. Patients with the history of recurrent significant pregnancy complications (ie, recurrent first or second trimester losses) may consider surgical treatment of endometriosis to mitigate risk in pregnancy when other options have failed. However, there is a significant paucity of evidence to support this indication for treatment, and thorough preoperative counseling of risks associated with endometriosis surgery must be reviewed.

*Clinical tip*
There is no evidence that surgical treatment of endometriosis before pregnancy will improve pregnancy outcomes and as a result is not an indication on its own.

*Additional surgical considerations*
Additional considerations exist that may inform the decision to pursue surgery. Individual religious and/or sociocultural backgrounds and financial situations may strongly influence fertility options. An open discussion between patient and provider is essential in the determination of what options are acceptable. Individual religions have varied views on the acceptability of different forms of ART.[44] Finally, government or insurance funding for ART is not universal and there may be significant financial barriers to the pursuit of fertility treatments. Therefore, surgery may be the only acceptable option.[45]

## Approach to Surgery: Intra-Operative Considerations

*Step 1: verify the goal of surgery*
The approach to surgical management of endometriosis begins with a thoughtful preoperative evaluation to determine the extent of expected disease, the impact on the patient (symptoms), and the goals of intervention. The personalized approach for endometriosis care is a patient-centered perspective, in contrast to the disease-centric viewpoint which would focus solely on disease eradication (**Fig. 4**). Ultimately the "goal" of surgery should consider each aspect and reduce the harm while maximizing the benefit to the patient.

*Step 2: surgical approaches*
When fertility preservation or optimization is considered, the surgical approach must be balanced with improving outcomes while managing the risk of harm. Essentially, any surgery for endometriosis is a complex balancing act between maximum disease management and sparing normal function and organs.

**Excision versus ablation.** Based on the data extracted from a recent systematic review and meta-analysis, no significant difference between laparoscopic excision and ablation was noted in regard to improving pain from minimal and mild endometriosis.[46] This discussion is limited to superficial disease as the management of DE cannot be managed by ablation alone. Excision of deep disease is best managed by those with expertise and appropriate skills to manage the retroperitoneum and adjacent organ involvement (bladder, bowel, ureter).

**Cystectomy versus ablation or electrocoagulation for endometriomas.** Damage to the ovary can occur at several steps during the surgical approach to an endometrioma, including removal of normal ovarian cortex containing follicles during ovarian dissection, and damage incurred while obtaining hemostasis. Several surgical techniques are proposed for the surgical management of endometriomas.

   In general, ovarian cystectomy or excision of the endometrioma is preferred over ablation or electrocoagulation as it is associated with a reduction in the recurrence of the endometrioma, long-term pain relief, and increase in spontaneous pregnancy rates.[25] However, the risk of harming ovarian reserve, as outlined above, should be considered. There has been a call to reconsider ablation of ovarian endometrioma in selected cases with carbon dioxide laser and plasma energy in cases of infertility.[47] This "conservative" approach addresses the goals of the patient, and if fertility is the priority, then the least harm with the best outcome should be the goal instead of complete and radical excision. Furthermore, among women who will subsequently

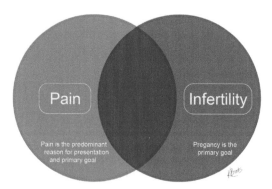

**Fig. 4.** Goal setting–pain, infertility, or both.

undergo fertility treatment after surgery for endometrioma, there is insufficient evidence to favor excisional surgery over ablative surgery.[48]

### Step 3: adhesion prevention

**Adhesion barriers.** At the completion of the procedure, anti-adhesions measures have been used in an attempt to reduce postoperative adhesion formation and when applicable place ovaries within the posterior cul-de-sac or close to the vaginal apex for ease of future transvaginal oocyte retrieval. However, there is no overwhelming data in the literature which supports any specific anti-adhesion material or intervention for pelvic surgery.[49] This is further complicated by the significant heterogeneity of the endometriosis presentation and surgical interventions. Novel interventions are ongoing and show promise, including a recent randomized control trial by Krämer and colleagues[50] demonstrating benefit at 2 months post endometriosis surgery of an anti-adhesion agent at second-look laparoscopy. Further research in this space is required before generalizability for all endometriosis surgical cases.

**Temporary ovarian suspension.** Ovarian adhesions to the sidewall or uterus are likely some of the most problematic adhesions among patients who are under surgery for endometriosis. Temporary ovarian suspension has been proposed as one method to prevent this scenario. The thought is that if the ovaries are lifted from the pelvic sidewall, bowel, or cul-de-sac, they may not adhere in the long term (**Fig. 5**A–C). This type of suspension has been described with suture tied outside the abdominal wall or with quickly dissolving intra-abdominal suture material. A systematic review on the topic by Giampaolino and colleagues demonstrated the potential positive outcomes of this intervention; however, further RCTs with larger sample sizes are required.[51] The concept and data are promising; however, still require larger studies with improved ultrasound experience to evaluate the impact on ovarian accessibility for oocyte retrieval.

### Step 4: know when to stop

The complete eradication of endometriosis has long been advocated among surgeons who focus on this disease process. Complete "excision" has been touted as the gold standard of care. For those with infertility or wishing to preserve fertility, this approach may lead to more harm than benefit. If a patient has no symptoms other than infertility, is it necessary to always perform aggressive visceral resection (especially in nonobstructive disease processes)? This fundamental question leads to the importance of the surgical team taking the step of intraoperative decision making to assist with patient care. In the ideal world, thorough evaluation with excellence in imaging would provide a complete preoperative plan for every patient. However, the reality is that

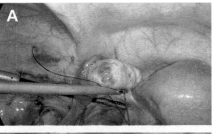
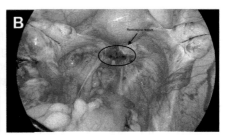
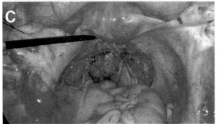

**Fig. 5.** (A) Temporary ovarian suspension (to external abdominal wall); (B) Facilitates exposure for managing deep endometriosis of the posterior compartment; (C) Temporary suspension sutures may be removed 24 to 72 hours later to theoretically prevent adhesions.

imaging is highly variable globally and the skill set of surgeons is also not uniformly established. As a result, it is important to identify one's limits as a surgeon and to establish a risk mitigation approach among patients whereby fertility is a priority. This honest and frank discussion with the patient and team is essential to reduce complications and optimize outcomes after surgery.

## SUMMARY

Determining the role of surgery for endometriosis among those with related infertility or those with future fertility goals can be challenging. Endometriosis has a wide variety of clinical and pathologic presentations which makes it almost impossible to have a single approach for all patients and this is further reflected by the lack of high-quality evidence to guide decision making. In general, for patients with endometriosis-related infertility who wish to achieve pregnancy, ART is preferred over surgery. However, a personalized approach to care is necessary, and a thorough history, physical examination, and imaging will help inform the decision for surgery and counseling regarding the risks and benefits of surgery. The patient with significant pain, risk of malignancy, or disease resulting in organ obstruction or dysfunction is best managed with surgical care by an experienced team including consultation with a fertility specialist. Surgery should be considered cautiously among patients whereby fertility is a priority, given the risk of postoperative adhesions and damage to ovarian reserve. The classic surgical perspective that dictates mandatory radical excision of "all endometriosis" may be better replaced by goal-directed surgical treatment of endometriosis in this population. If the goal is pregnancy in the future, then surgical care should enhance that outcome when possible.

## ACKNOWLEDGMENTS

The authors would like to thank Kaylee C. L. Brooks, PhD Candidate (University of Ottawa) for the adapted and original illustrations and graphic design work in this article.

## DISCLOSURE

Dr J. Gale is supported by a Departmental Research Grant Award through her institution. Dr S.S. Singh has received research grants (through his institution), participated in advisory boards, and created and presented CME sessions for Abbvie and Bayer. He has also received honoraria for CME sessions with Myovant and Hologic.

## REFERENCES

1. Tomassetti C, Johnson NP, Petrozza J, et al. An international terminology for endometriosis, 2021. Hum Reprod Open 2021;4:hoab029. Oct 22;2021.
2. Zondervan KT, Becker CM, Koga K, et al. Endometriosis. Nat Rev Dis Primer 2018;4(1):1–25.
3. Viganò P, Parazzini F, Somigliana E, et al. Endometriosis: epidemiology and aetiological factors. Best Pract Res Clin Obstet Gynaecol 2004;18(2):177–200.
4. Lin Y-H, Chen Y-H, Chang H-Y, et al. Chronic niche inflammation in endometriosis-associated infertility: current understanding and future therapeutic strategies. Int J Mol Sci 2018;19(8):2385.
5. Endometriosis and infertility: a committee opinion. Fertil Steril 2012;98(3):591–8.
6. American Society for Reproductive. Revised american society for reproductive medicine classification of endometriosis: 1996. Fertil Steril 1997;67(5):817–21.
7. International working group of AAGL, ESGE, ESHRE and WES, Vermeulen N, Abrao MS, Einarsson JI, et al. Endometriosis classification, staging and reporting systems: a review on the road to a universally accepted endometriosis classification. Hum Reprod Open 2021;2021(4):hoab025.
8. Abrao MS, Andres MP, Miller CE, et al. AAGL 2021 endometriosis classification: an anatomy-based surgical complexity score. J Minim Invasive Gynecol 2021; 28(11):1941–50.e1.
9. Adamson GD, Pasta DJ. Endometriosis fertility index: the new, validated endometriosis staging system. Fertil Steril 2010;94(5):1609–15.
10. Tomassetti C, Bafort C, Meuleman C, et al. Reproducibility of the endometriosis fertility index: a prospective inter-/intra-rater agreement study. BJOG 2020; 127(1):107–14.
11. Vesali S, Razavi M, Rezaeinejad M, et al. Endometriosis fertility index for predicting non-assisted reproductive technology pregnancy after endometriosis surgery: a systematic review and meta-analysis. BJOG 2020;127(7):800–9.
12. Vilasagar S, Bougie O, Singh SS. A practical guide to the clinical evaluation of endometriosis-associated pelvic pain. J Minim Invasive Gynecol 2020;27(2): 270–9.
13. Young SW, Groszmann Y, Dahiya N, et al. Sonographer-acquired ultrasound protocol for deep endometriosis. Abdom Radiol(NY) 2020;45(6):1659–69.
14. Fraser MA, Agarwal S, Chen I, et al. Routine vs. expert-guided transvaginal ultrasound in the diagnosis of endometriosis: A retrospective review. Abdom Imaging 2015;40(3):587–94.
15. Guerriero S, Condous G, van den Bosch T, et al. Systematic approach to sonographic evaluation of the pelvis in women with suspected endometriosis, including terms, definitions and measurements: a consensus opinion from the international deep endometriosis analysis (IDEA) group. Ultrasound Obstet Gynecol 2016;48(3):318–32.
16. Tong A, VanBuren WM, Chamié L, et al. Recommendations for MRI technique in the evaluation of pelvic endometriosis: consensus statement from the society of

abdominal radiology endometriosis disease-focused panel. Abdom Radiol(NY) 2020;45(6):1569–86.

17. Volodarsky-Perel A, Buckett W, Tulandi T. Treatment of hydrosalpinx in relation to IVF outcome: a systematic review and meta-analysis. Reprod Biomed Online 2019;39(3):413–32.

18. Somigliana E, Benaglia L, Paffoni A, et al. Risks of conservative management in women with ovarian endometriomas undergoing IVF. Hum Reprod Update 2015; 21(4):486–99.

19. Marcoux S, Maheux R, Bérubé S. Laparoscopic surgery in infertile women with minimal or mild endometriosis. canadian collaborative group on endometriosis. N Engl J Med 1997;337(4):217–22.

20. Parazzini F. Ablation of lesions or no treatment in minimal-mild endometriosis in infertile women: a randomized trial. gruppo italiano per lo studio dell'endometriosi. Hum Reprod 1999;14(5):1332–4.

21. Busacca M, Vignali M. Ovarian endometriosis: from pathogenesis to surgical treatment. Curr Opin Obstet Gynecol 2003;15(4):321–6.

22. Redwine DB. Ovarian endometriosis: a marker for more extensive pelvic and intestinal disease. Fertil Steril 1999;72(2):310–5.

23. Chapron C, Pietin-Vialle C, Borghese B, et al. Associated ovarian endometrioma is a marker for greater severity of deeply infiltrating endometriosis. Fertil Steril 2009;92(2):453–7.

24. Dunselman GAJ, Vermeulen N, Becker C, et al. ESHRE guideline: management of women with endometriosis. Hum Reprod 2014;29(3):400–12.

25. Hart RJ, Hickey M, Maouris P, Buckett W. Excisional surgery versus ablative surgery for ovarian endometriomata. Cochrane Database of Systematic Reviews 2008;(2). https://doi.org/10.1002/14651858.CD004992.pub3. Art. No.: CD004992.

26. Garcia-Velasco JA, Somigliana E. Management of endometriomas in women requiring IVF: to touch or not to touch. Hum Reprod 2008;24(3):496–501.

27. Cranney R, Condous G, Reid S. An update on the diagnosis, surgical management, and fertility outcomes for women with endometrioma. Acta Obstet Gynecol Scand 2017;96(6):633–43.

28. Benschop L, Farquhar C, van der Poel N, Heineman MJ. Interventions for women with endometrioma prior to assisted reproductive technology. Cochrane Database of Systematic Reviews 2010;(11). https://doi.org/10.1002/14651858.CD008571.pub2. Art. No.: CD008571.

29. Karadağ C, Yoldemir T, Demircan Karadağ S, et al. The effects of endometrioma size and bilaterality on ovarian reserve. J Obstet Gynaecol 2020;40(4):531–6.

30. Alammari R, Lightfoot M, Hur H-C. Impact of cystectomy on ovarian reserve: review of the literature. J Minim Invasive Gynecol 2017;24(2):247–57.

31. Busacca M, Riparini J, Somigliana E, et al. Postsurgical ovarian failure after laparoscopic excision of bilateral endometriomas. Am J Obstet Gynecol 2006;195(2):421–5.

32. Guo S-W. Recurrence of endometriosis and its control. Hum Reprod Update 2009;15(4):441–61.

33. Vercellini P, Somigliana E, Daguati R, et al. Postoperative oral contraceptive exposure and risk of endometrioma recurrence. Am J Obstet Gynecol 2008;198(5):504.e1–5.

34. Muzii L, Tucci CD, Achilli C, et al. Continuous versus cyclic oral contraceptives after laparoscopic excision of ovarian endometriomas: a systematic review and metaanalysis. Am J Obstet Gynecol 2016;214(2):203–11.

35. Fauconnier A, Chapron C, Dubuisson J-B, et al. Relation between pain symptoms and the anatomic location of deep infiltrating endometriosis. Fertil Steril 2002; 78(4):719–26.
36. Iversen ML, Seyer-Hansen M, Forman A. Does surgery for deep infiltrating bowel endometriosis improve fertility? a systematic review. Acta Obstet Gynecol Scand 2017;96(6):688–93.
37. Casals G, Carrera M, Domínguez JA, et al. Impact of surgery for deep infiltrative endometriosis before in vitro fertilization: a systematic review and meta-analysis. J Minim Invasive Gynecol 2021;28(7):1303–12, e5.
38. Berlanda N, Vercellini P, Somigliana E, et al. Role of Surgery in Endometriosis-Associated Subfertility. Semin Reprod Med 2013;31(2):133–43.
39. Vercellini P, Barbara G, Abbiati A, et al. Repetitive surgery for recurrent symptomatic endometriosis: what to do? Eur J Obstet Gynecol Reprod Biol 2009;146(1): 15–21.
40. Abrao MS, Petraglia F, Falcone T, et al. Deep endometriosis infiltrating the rectosigmoid: critical factors to consider before management. Hum Reprod Update 2015;21(3):329–39.
41. Jago CA, Nguyen DB, Flaxman TE, et al. Bowel surgery for endometriosis: A practical look at short- and long-term complications. Best Pract Res Clin Obstet Gynaecol 2021;71:144–60.
42. Soriano D, Adler I, Bouaziz J, et al. Fertility outcome of laparoscopic treatment in patients with severe endometriosis and repeated in vitro fertilization failures. Fertil Steril 2016;106(5):1264–9.
43. Chen I, Lalani S, Xie R, et al. Association between surgically diagnosed endometriosis and adverse pregnancy outcomes. Fertil Steril 2018;109(1):142–7.
44. Schenker J g. Women's reproductive health: monotheistic religious perspectives. Int J Gynecol Obstet 2000;70(1):77–86.
45. Singh SS, Suen MWH. Surgery for endometriosis: beyond medical therapies. Fertil Steril 2017;107(3):549–54.
46. Burks C, Lee M, DeSarno M, et al. Excision versus ablation for management of minimal to mild endometriosis: a systematic review and meta-analysis. J Minim Invasive Gynecol 2021;28(3):587–97.
47. Darwish B, Roman H. When opportunity knocks, grab your chance: shall ablation be rehabilitated in the treatment of endometrioma? J Minim Invasive Gynecol 2021;28(1):1–2.
48. Candiani M, Ferrari S, Bartiromo L, et al. Fertility outcome after co2 laser vaporization versus cystectomy in women with ovarian endometrioma: a comparative study. J Minim Invasive Gynecol 2021;28(1):34–41.
49. Ahmad G, Kim K, Thompson M, et al. Barrier agents for adhesion prevention after gynaecological surgery. Cochrane Database Syst Rev 2020;3:CD000475.
50. Krämer B, Andress J, Neis F, et al. Adhesion prevention after endometriosis surgery — results of a randomized, controlled clinical trial with second-look laparoscopy. Langenbecks Arch Surg 2021;406(6):2133–43.
51. Giampaolino P, Corte LD, Saccone G, et al. Role of ovarian suspension in preventing postsurgical ovarian adhesions in patients with stage III-IV pelvic endometriosis: a systematic review. J Minim Invasive Gynecol 2019;26(1):53–62.

# Hysterectomy for Chronic Pelvic Pain

Richard Cockrum, MD[a,b], Frank Tu, MD, MPH[a,b],*

## KEYWORDS

- Hysterectomy • Chronic pelvic pain • Surgical treatment
- Perioperative management

## KEY POINTS

- Hysterectomy for chronic pelvic pain (CPP) is likely most effective when symptoms are linked to menstrual pain, menstrual activity, and a reproducibly tender uterus on examination.
- Patients with CPP are more likely to have chronic overlapping pain conditions (COPCs) and to require multi-modal therapies for optimal results. These conditions do not preclude hysterectomy as a treatment of targeted symptoms.
- The few available studies of hysterectomy report favorable outcomes for pelvic pain in well selected patients, with only 5% to 26% of cases failing to result in significant or complete improvement. However, 38% of patients without pathologic abnormalities reported persistent pelvic pain after 12 months in one study.
- Identifying COPCs and psychological risk factors for chronic pain can inform perioperative management with the goal to improve short-term recovery and decrease risk of persistent pain after hysterectomy.

## INTRODUCTION

Chronic pelvic pain (CPP) has an estimated prevalence of 15% in the adult female population of the US and has been estimated to be the primary reason for 4% to 12% of all hysterectomies for benign indications.[1–3] More recent and specific data are not available from epidemiologic studies because CPP is poorly captured by administrative claims data and due to lack of a singular, widely used definition of CPP, which continues to be debated.[4]

Several clinical practice guidelines have addressed surgical management options for CPP.[5] The level and grade of evidence cited varies, but most recommend hysterectomy for severe or refractory symptoms. The 2020 clinical guideline by the American

[a] Department of Obstetrics and Gynecology, NorthShore University HealthSystem, Walgreen's Bldg 1507, 2650 Ridge Avenue, Evanston, IL 60201, USA; [b] Department of Obstetrics and Gynecology, University of Chicago, Pritzker School of Medicine, Chicago, IL, USA
* Corresponding author.
*E-mail address:* ftu@northshore.org

Obstet Gynecol Clin N Am 49 (2022) 257–271
https://doi.org/10.1016/j.ogc.2022.02.008
0889-8545/22/© 2022 Elsevier Inc. All rights reserved.

College of Obstetricians and Gynecologists (ACOG) on the evaluation and management of CPP does not address the efficacy, effectiveness, or best practices for hysterectomy.[6] However, this major surgery remains an important option even as cases annually are overall decreasing due to improved conservative management for leiomyomas and endometriosis.

In this narrative review, we examine 4 essential issues for the gynecologic surgeon considering hysterectomy for a patient with CPP:

1. Conceptual framework underlying hysterectomy as a treatment modality for patients with CPP;
2. Long-term outcomes demonstrating the efficacy of hysterectomy for patients with CPP;
3. Optimizing individualized benefits and risks of surgery through preoperative assessment and counseling; and
4. Perioperative care for the patient undergoing hysterectomy for CPP.

## DISCUSSION
### Section 1: conceptual framework

For the practicing clinician, we lead with an overarching view of this topic. Based on our clinical experience and read of the literature, hysterectomy for CPP is likely most effective, with durable results, when there is clearly a major component of the patient's symptoms linked to menstrual pain or menstrual activity. Further, hysterectomy is likely to be successful if the dominant feature of the evaluation is a reproducibly tender uterus on pelvic examination.

Some clinicians do not count leiomyoma, advanced endometriosis, or diffuse adenomyosis as CPP conditions when these are the dominant source of pain. When presenting in isolation, these conditions seem to respond well to hysterectomy. In our experience, we have similar success in hysterectomy for chronic uterine pain without visible pathology following persistently symptomatic dysmenorrhea or following acute uterine irritation (eg, intrauterine device insertion, endometrial ablation with or without tubal sterilization, pelvic inflammatory disease). These specific etiologies have not been covered in published CPP hysterectomy case series and observational cohorts.[7] Consistent success for symptom relief of chronic uterine pain is less predictable if:

- Only minor uterine pathology is present (eg, incidental small leiomyoma, random islands of adenomyosis)
- Tenderness on examination poorly or incompletely reproduces the primary pain symptoms
- Minimal dysmenorrhea is present
- Multiple chronic overlapping pain conditions (COPCs) are present (eg, IBS, bladder pain syndrome [BPS]/interstitial cystitis [IC])
- Pain is widespread throughout the abdomen and pelvis
- Psychological comorbidity such as depression significantly impairs quality of life
- Central sensory sensitivity is evident by clinical assessment or as measured by scales such as the Fibromyalgia Survey Score (FSS)

The presence of multiple COPCs in a woman presenting with CPP should raise concerns for a gynecologist that separate from any peripheral pelvic pathology, she may also have dysregulations in central nervous system pathways involved in threat appraisal. This neurocognitive processing dysfunction leads to the abnormal interpretation of peripheral afferent signaling from abdominopelvic tissues (eg, bladder, bowel, pelvic floor) that may not readily resolve with removal of the uterus.[8,9] The underlying mechanisms may include alterations in the activity of spinal interneurons, connections between different cortical centers, and impaired descending modulation.[10] On the other hand, pain symptoms may also be exacerbated by cross-organ sensitization, a well-known process underlying some CPP cases.

In particular, severe undertreated dysmenorrhea at menarche seems to predispose patients to developing CPP outside the uterus. Some women with that history may find further resolution of bowel or bladder complaints after their hysterectomy as an unexpected side benefit. As a corollary to this concept, postoperative recovery must be well managed for patients with multiple COPCs so that a new potential pain generator does not emerge, either a discrete organ-based syndrome or chronic postsurgical pain. For patients with a mixed presentation of chronic pain conditions, predicting who will have a significant improvement after hysterectomy remains a critical research question.

### Section 2: Long-Term Outcomes

Measurement of the efficacy of hysterectomy for CPP has long been plagued by ambiguous research definitions. Most studies have not carefully defined patients with preoperative pelvic pain with the same criteria used for CPP. Comparisons between studies have been further limited by heterogenous data on postoperative outcomes: persistent pelvic pain (undefined), persistent CPP, chronic postsurgical pain, functional outcomes (eg, return to normal activity, sexual activity, and bladder and bowel function), and need for additional surgery.[11]

### Early studies on persistent chronic pelvic pain

The literature on the effectiveness of hysterectomy for CPP conditions has largely come from smaller, single-site, observational studies. In 1990, Stovall and colleagues published the first data on long-term outcomes: a retrospective case-control study of 99 patients undergoing hysterectomy for presumed uterine etiology for CPP (with exclusions for extrauterine disease and uterine weight >200g at the time of surgery).[12] Nearly all women reported dysmenorrhea (94%) and had uterine tenderness (97%). Resolution of pain occurred in 78% (77/99) women at an average of 21.6 months of follow-up. Of the remainder, 17 patients reported partial improvement, and 5 patients reported worse pain than before surgery. Details on the character or etiology of persistent CPP were not mentioned. Differences in symptomatology, hysterectomy route, concomitant procedures, or uterine pathology did not predict the success of surgery. On pathologic review, 66% of patients had a normal uterus.

In 1995, Hillis and colleagues published the first multi-center prospective observational cohort study on persistent CPP after total abdominal hysterectomy.[13] Among 308 women with CPP as the primary indication for hysterectomy, 74% of patients reported complete resolution of pain at 1-year follow-up and 21% reported persistent but decreased pain. Consistent with the prior study, 5% of patients reported no change or worsening pain. Though an absence of identifiable pelvic pathology doubled the odds of persistent CPP, 62% of patients in this subgroup were pain-free 1 year after surgery.

Variable but favorable pain responses have been described in 2 earlier studies. Carlson and colleagues reported some degree of continued preoperative pelvic pain in 5% (14/273) of patients at 1 year of follow-up.[14] In a cross-sectional study of women with a primary surgical indication of pelvic pain, Tay and Bromwich found that 96% (94/98) of women at 1 year following total abdominal hysterectomy had partial (18%) or complete (78%) improvement.[15]

### Persistent chronic pelvic pain and neuropsychological factors

More recent work has extended these initial outcome measures to understand what other psychological or neurologic factors may predict clinical response to hysterectomy, as these are core aspects of chronic pain syndromes. The challenge with those studies is the inclusion of heterogeneous populations of patients without all having a consistent formal diagnosis for CPP.

Regarding the presence of comorbid depression, Hartmann and colleagues in 2004 studied 1249 women from the Maryland Hysterectomy multisite study to characterize how depression and preoperative pain levels predict postoperative persistent CPP and functional outcomes.[16] While 32% of women met their criteria for CPP (moderate to severe levels for 14 days in the last month), only 1% had pain as the primary indication for hysterectomy.

In that study, having preoperative pelvic pain incurred a 2.22 higher odds of reporting a pelvic pain problem at 24 months, while having comorbid depression and pelvic pain had a 4.91 increased odds. However, the absolute reduction in reported pelvic pain was striking—with reductions in those 2 groups from 95% to 97% preoperatively to only 9% to 19% at 24 months postoperatively. Similarly, large improvements in physical and mental health (using the Medical Outcome Study Short-Form General Health Survey) were seen following hysterectomy even among the self-identified pelvic pain patients.

As a well-established feature of chronic pain syndromes, central sensory sensitivity is a known risk factor for higher use of opioids postoperatively and for the development of new-onset chronic postsurgical pain. A study published in 2021 by As-Sanie et al. assessed the impact of broad central sensory sensitivity (using the 31 point Fibromyalgia Survey Scale [FSS]) on persistent pelvic pain at 6 months after hysterectomy.[17] Out of 126 women studied, 24% had CPP as an indication for hysterectomy, and review of pathology and operative reports indicated a heterogeneous group: 51% leiomyoma, 46% adenomyosis, 15% endometriosis. These women reported a substantial baseline average pelvic pain, which was not significantly different between those without persistent pelvic pain compared with those with persistent pelvic pain (5.3/10 vs 6.1/10, $P = 10$). Most women (111/126%, 88%) achieved the primary specified outcome: at least a 50% improvement from baseline pelvic pain. Among the 15 (12%) cases defined as failures, only 5 (4%) women reported persistent or worsening pain.

In a multivariable regression model, baseline central sensory sensitivity profile significantly predicted the likelihood of persistent pelvic pain status (OR: 1.27 [95% CI: 1.03–1.58], for each point increase on FSS) and absolute pain score. However, 95% of women in the highest FSS tertile still managed to achieve a pelvic pain score less than or equal to 1.8/10 at 6 months. This remarkable improvement in a group at high risk for persistent pain supported the main conclusions by the study authors. Central sensory sensitivity and other risk factors should not limit the potential benefit of hysterectomy to treat a peripheral pain generator as identified by history and examination, Instead, assessments like the FSS can be used to inform counseling on postoperative outcomes and planning for additional perioperative management strategies that target central sensory sensitivity (examples reviewed later in this article). In contrast to the prior literature, depression, anxiety, severity and duration of preoperative pain, history of endometriosis, or hysterectomy route (almost all laparoscopic or vaginal) were not associated with postoperative outcomes in the combined predictive model.

Collectively, both studies, one done in a broad community setting by Hartmann and colleagues, and one done in a tertiary pelvic pain referral clinic setting by As-Sanie et al., suggest that despite comorbid psychological issues or sensory sensitivity, a large proportion of patients with baseline CPP will achieve significant relief from hysterectomy. Future studies would benefit from a careful appraisal of how clinical examination findings might help predict the potential benefit of hysterectomy.

## Section 3: Optimizing Individualized Benefits and Risks of Surgery

### Predicting success: history, examination, and imaging
The easier recovery from the widely used laparoscopic approach may bias women and their clinicians to view hysterectomy as the panacea for nonspecific pelvic pain. To inform proper preoperative assessment, case selection, and counseling, clinicians should perform a targeted history, careful examination, and ordering/review of imaging.

We cannot overemphasize the importance of exploring a patient's general history of pain before focusing on reproductive organs and tissues. Intuitively, severe midline pain largely resembling symptoms of dysmenorrhea, but throughout the month, is more likely to reflect a primary uterine source of pain compared with noncyclic pain of another location or character. In contrast, identifying symptoms suggestive of IBS, BPS/ IC, myofascial pelvic pain (MPP), or a broad swath of COPCs may reduce the potential for hysterectomy to effectively treat pelvic pain.

Awareness of prior trauma experiences, which are present in over 40% of women with CPP in tertiary referral clinics,[18] will also help prepare the patient for the possibility of a more complex pain response postoperatively, or of having latent chronic pain conditions unmasked. Understanding which analgesics and adjuvant medications (eg, neuromodulators) have been effective previously, location of prior pathology, and prior surgical approaches used may minimize intraoperative complications and poor postoperative pain control. A patient desiring future fertility will naturally not be a candidate for hysterectomy, but a small minority of nulliparous women with recalcitrant symptoms may nonetheless opt for this approach.

We use a systematic approach to the physical examination for all patients with CPP regardless of where they are in the therapeutic journey. Because symptoms of COPCs may wax and wane over time, the examination should be repeated preoperatively to confirm the uterus remains tender and to account for any meaningful untreated pain generators. There are also obvious features such as focal symptoms that will suggest the value of precise examination maneuvers to detect the presence of deep infiltrating endometriosis or nerve entrapment. These conditions are important to consider, as they might respond sufficiently to conservative therapy. As part of a standardized and comprehensive examination (similar to one reported by Abu-Alnadi et al.[19]), we recommend special attention to the following:

- Abdominal wall: inspection for prior surgical scars as sites of possible nerve injury
- Abdominal wall: Carnett's sign to aid in differentiating pain from the abdominal wall and viscera or other internal pain
- Single-digit vaginal examination: palpate Alcock's canal to identify pudendal neuropathy
- Single-digit vaginal examination: assess muscles (eg, levator ani, obturator internus) for tone and tenderness—noting if palpation recreates the primary pain complaint, dyspareunia, or neither
- Bimanual examination (preferably with a single internally inserted digit): gentle palpation of the urogenital structures, rectovaginal septum, uterosacral ligaments, uterus, and adnexa—noting any restriction in mobility and attempting to isolate sensitivity of adjacent structures

Separate from hysterectomy planning, preoperative evaluation of the patient with CPP mandates imaging, typically a pelvic ultrasound. This information is generally available ahead of any counseling about surgical success rates. Diagnosis of uterine pathology (eg, leiomyoma, adenomyoma, adenomyosis) can complement examination findings for the attribution of chronic pain to a distinct, focal source; however, most definitions of CPP typically exclude the diagnosis of a structural abnormality as the root cause. Separately, imaging may detect a nonuterine cause of pelvic pain that might not respond to hysterectomy alone, such as deep infiltrating endometriosis in the rectovaginal septum or occult adnexal pathology that might need preoperative evaluation.

One other imaging consideration is pelvic venography, which has been suggested to evaluate for the incompetence of the pelvic veins promoting blood flow stasis, inflammation, and nerve activation—known as pelvic congestion syndrome. The diagnostic accuracy of such studies has never been carefully studied, and findings of enlarged ovarian veins, varicosities, or delayed venous return can be found in significant numbers of asymptomatic women. Moreover, the symptom complex and physical examination findings purported to define this syndrome also have never been validated. Nonetheless, in one small RCT, women meeting the criteria for pelvic congestion syndrome reported a significant improvement in pain after hysterectomy and bilateral salpingo-oophorectomy.[20]

### Preoperative counseling for patients with chronic overlapping pain conditions

Each CPP case with a uterine pain component will present somewhat uniquely. Some patients are conveniently present with comorbid gynecologic symptoms or an antecedent history that may more predictably respond to hysterectomy: midline pelvic pain with abnormal uterine bleeding, postablation syndrome, or chronic gynecologic infections. Other presentations without specific gynecologic symptoms (eg, pelvic pain without concomitant menstrual bleeding issues or bulk symptoms, isolated deep dyspareunia without any evidence of pain on uterine or forniceal palpation, intermittent cramping with concurrent bowel dysfunction) require a caveat that their symptoms may not originate from the uterus even if the patient is convinced of its source. Complete details of symptomatology have not been captured in prior studies, so the frequency of these pain characteristics remains unknown.

We counsel patients that there is Level III evidence of high rates of persistent pain relief for endometriosis-associated pelvic pain without (77%) or with bilateral oophorectomy (92%) based on a case series by Shakiba and colleagues with 7 years of follow-up (n = 97 women).[21] Coexisting deep infiltrating endometriosis should be targeted at the same time, based on symptoms; however, not all cases of bowel endometriosis need excision, which again should be driven by the exact examination findings, particularly if the patient is interested in hormonal suppression postoperatively or if she is near menopause.

However, a patient who also reports prolonged, severe MPP or BPS/IC, will likely still follow the uncertain trajectory of those extrauterine conditions and require targeted therapy for those organs. For example, Chung and colleagues reported a case series of 111 women with CPP after hysterectomy whereby 79% were diagnosed with BPS/IC.[22] This cohort is illustrative of the challenge in treating CPP, as only a minority had improvement in pain with recommended therapies. Similar caveats should be given for severe midcycle pain or IBS. Patients with fibromyalgia or diffuse pain are a special case, and we strongly advise engagement in inter-disciplinary and multimodal care before surgery if possible.

Abu-Alnadi et al. have recently reported the first study to assess the prevalence of MPP before laparoscopic hysterectomy including those with and without CPP.[19] MPP was identified on standardized preoperative examination of the pelvic floor in 151/353 (43%) women, notably at a CPP referral center. It was strongly correlated with other chronic pain conditions (eg, low back pain, fibromyalgia) and worse short-term postoperative pain: 37% of patients with MPP reported pain of 5/10 or greater at 3 to 6 weeks compared with 1% of patients without MPP. In our practice, we advise patients with abdominal and pelvic myofascial pain that they may experience increased pain in the immediate postoperative period and offer pelvic floor physical therapy referral and muscle relaxants for use before and after surgery. Similar system-focused management should be considered for other COPCs previously discussed.

### Risks of surgery

Patients requesting hysterectomy for CPP treatment may be quite familiar with surgical recovery and risks, but a thorough review of those prior experiences and anticipated complications can optimize recovery and satisfaction. Because many of these patients will have CNS alterations consistent with central sensory sensitivity, it is important to look for and treat complications early. For example, suspected nerve entrapment, whether from abdominal wall or pelvic nerves if a deeper dissection or sacrospinous suspension is performed, respectively, deserves early treatment efforts with nerve injections, physical therapy, or early consideration of removal of sutures if the pain does not steadily improve . We also counsel patients about the rare complication of new vaginal cuff pain, which may poorly respond to medical and surgical interventions.[23]

The actual risk of de novo posthysterectomy pain is not well characterized in most prior studies as many hysterectomy patients have preoperative pain, even if CPP is not the indication for surgery. A large Danish study estimated chronic postsurgical pain occurs in up to 32% of patients, and a smaller prospective follow-up study suggested perhaps half of those women have some degree of significant pain.[3,24] Benolo and colleagues reported a recent prospective cohort at 12 weeks postoperatively whereby 32% of patients reported any pain, but only 6% reported moderate to severe pain (4/10 or greater).[25]

Finally, as CPP is typically a condition of reproductive age women, women should be counseled about the risk of regret from hysterectomy, which has a durable 1-year estimate of about 7% based on the Detroit Hysterectomy Regret study.[26] The predictor of such regret primarily was lack of initial satisfaction with the decision to have this surgery, supporting the need to elicit patient engagement thoroughly in such planning.

### Concurrent procedures

Perhaps the most important surgical planning question for hysterectomy for patients with CPP is whether to conserve the ovaries. In our experience, a well-counseled, premenopausal patient with CPP will almost always opt for retention even when advised about the 13% higher reoperation risk over 7 years for endometriosis-associated pelvic pain.[21] The known reduction in lifespan with early oophorectomy without hormone replacement (especially before age 40–45) and the concerns about small risks of hormone replacement therapy (eg, acute side effects, venous thromboembolism) seem to be strong drivers of that preference.[27] Notably, reoperation for oophorectomy has been shown to improve pelvic pain at short-term follow-up in 60% of carefully selected patients but with complication rates similar to laparoscopic hysterectomy.[28] If there is strong concern that the ovaries may be scarred down and cause recurrence of pain due to severe cul-de-sac disease, one option is to consider an oophoropexy with permanent suture up to the side wall.

If oophorectomy is planned, careful attention is needed to avoid leaving a remnant behind that may cause persistent CPP. Behera and colleagues reported on a case series (n = 124 women) with CPP after hysterectomy and bilateral salpingo-oophorectomy who underwent laparoscopic evaluation.[29] The most common indications for the index surgery were endometriosis (45%) and CPP (20%), and the most prevalent findings at subsequent laparoscopy were adhesions (94%), endometriosis (15%), and ovarian remnants (26%). Concurrent ovarian remnant and endometriosis were found in 10 (8%) patients. For women found to have ovarian remnant syndrome, 70% reported improvement postoperatively, highlighting the importance of prevention through excellent surgical technique at the index surgery. When the ovaries are adherent to the side wall, additional preventative steps may include ureterolysis and ensuring an adequate margin in excision of peritoneum and transection of the infundibulopelvic ligament.

As previously discussed, deeply infiltrating endometriosis should be addressed if it can be reasonably linked to the symptom presentation. However, in our experience, old fibrosis in the side wall does not necessitate a broad peritonectomy in search of "complete excision" when the primary indication is the treatment of uterine pain (by examination and symptoms).

### Section 4: Perioperative Care

Once the decision for hysterectomy is made, there are numerous opportunities to improve the patient's perioperative experience and surgical outcomes. A comprehensive review of Enhanced Recovery After Surgery (ERAS) protocols has been recently published in a white paper from the AAGL.[30] Urinary retention, nausea, and uncontrolled pain are the most significant barriers to achieving same-day discharge in medically healthy patients.[31] Accordingly, patients with CPP often have multiple risk factors for failed same-day discharge. Setting expectations may be the most important and modifiable, albeit challenging, step in optimizing postoperative recovery for patients with CPP. We highlight key considerations for patients with CPP from ERAS components and evidence from the broader chronic pain literature.

#### Preoperative opioid, opioid agonist/antagonist, benzodiazepine, and substance use

For patient's using chronic opioids under a pain contract, we recommend contacting that provider directly to confirm the plan for multi-modal perioperative pain management and to establish who will prescribe postoperative opioids. Additional opioids should be prescribed above preoperative levels. It may be helpful for the patient to complete an anesthesiology preoperative visit to discuss options like ketamine or lidocaine infusions, or regional anesthesia. These have not been shown to improve pain and recovery outcomes in the general laparoscopic hysterectomy population, but studies have not specifically assessed patients with CPP.[30] At our institution, we recommend an opioid taper (eg, goal of 20 morphine milligram equivalents [MME] per day) 1 to 2 weeks before surgery in an effort to improve postoperative response to opioids. However, this is not recommended by some others.[30]

For patients with baseline benzodiazepine, alcohol, or other drug use, careful instruction should be provided on risks of severe sedation or respiratory depression. Cessation of tobacco and heavy alcohol use at least 4 weeks before surgery is recommended.[30] Many organizations recommend prescribing naloxone for patients using concomitant opioids and benzodiazepines or high dose opioids alone (>50 MME per day).[32] We also warn patients using both opioids and gabapentinoids, an important class of adjuvant medications for patients with chronic pain, that increased side effects including respiratory depression have been reported.

### Postoperative care for patients with chronic pain

Patients with chronic pain experience higher levels of postoperative pain after hysterectomy and have a decreased response to analgesics.[33] Catastrophizing and other psychological risk factors such as anxiety and depression may contribute to this relationship. Ideally, patients with these risk factors would engage with an interdisciplinary treatment team before hysterectomy, including a therapist experienced with chronic pain. Laying this groundwork for patients experiencing acute postoperative pain is challenging, but focused interventions may be translatable for the perioperative team (eg, surgeon, nursing, primary care provider).

Postoperative outcomes may be improved through nonpharmacological interventions including physical, psychological, or both.[34] Depending on the case and timeline to surgery, these options may be initiated pre or postoperatively. For example, pelvic floor physical therapy may improve myofascial hypertonicity with connective tissue release and build resiliency through pain biology education and mindfulness exercises.[35] Psychosocial support programs may be pursued through traditional means (eg, cognitive behavioral therapy, nursing-led coaching sessions) or convenient mobile and web-based platforms (eg, Curable Health, SuperBetter, Headspace).

Weinrib and colleagues have reviewed their approach for the Transitional Pain Service at Toronto General Hospital.[36] Their comprehensive program designed to support psychological flexibility in managing pain aims to improve acute postoperative pain, hasten functional recovery, and promote protective factors against chronic postsurgical pain. In **Table 1**, we match the theoretic framework by Weinrib and colleagues for 6 key psychological barriers to recovery with examples of postoperative challenges and supportive care approaches. Surgeons may find these tips most helpful for patients with previously described risk factors. Further research should investigate how multi-modal perioperative programs combining psychological and physical interventions may synergistically improve outcomes, similar to nonsurgical chronic pain treatment plans.

### Analgesics and adjuvants

Contemporary postoperative regimens use nonsteroidal anti-inflammatory drugs (NSAIDs) and acetaminophen with as-needed use of opioids or partial opioid agonists. In our experience, most patients with chronic pain do well with the same medications as patients without chronic pain, noting special prescribing considerations for patients with preoperative opioid or other high-risk medication use described previously. As-Sanie et al. and Wong and colleagues have both explored preoperative assessments to aid in the prediction of postoperative opioid use through the FSS and the Postoperative Opioid Calculator for Hysterectomy (POOCH), respectively.[33,37] The primary findings from these studies and the broader surgical literature is that patients have been prescribed 2 to 4 times the average number of opioid tablets actually used after hysterectomy. Strategies to reduce unused opioids include standardized prescribing guidelines with fewer tablets (eg, Michigan Surgical Quality Collaborative) and engaging patients in shared decision-making.[38] We tailor preoperative counseling and postoperative reassurance acknowledging that prolonged use of analgesics is often necessary for patients with chronic pain. While the POOCH does not perfectly predict postoperative opioid use, it highlights key risk factors for increased use that the surgeon should consider:

**Table 1**
Psychological barriers and example interventions to improve postoperative recovery for patients with chronic pain

| Barrier to Psychological Flexibility[a] | Postoperative Scenario | Examples of Supportive Care Reflecting Principles of Cognitive Behavioral Therapy (CBT)[b] |
|---|---|---|
| Inflexible Attention | Fixation on pain sensation impairs the ability to engage in other thoughts/the present. "All I can think about is how much pain I am in." | Suggest or guide the patient in activities to engage the 5 senses (eg, mindful eating, diaphragmatic breathing, body scan) and movement (eg, yoga). |
| Lack of Clarity Regarding Values and Direction | Depressed mood and pessimism about recovery trajectory predominate future thinking. "I'll never be able to make it through this." | Identify patient's values for recovery and highlight their strengths (intrinsic) and resources (extrinsic) to help them progress despite challenges. |
| Inactivity and Behavioral Avoidance | Pain sensation and pain catastrophizing slow or prevent the gradual resumption of daily activities and progress in other important functional domains. "I'm stuck where I am - no better off today than last week." | Advise using a journal to track progress toward functional capacity while acknowledging that this work may temporarily increase sensations of pain and distress. It is critical for the patient and their support system and/or care team to celebrate small successes. |
| Self-as-Content | Inability to separate emotions and automatic thoughts from actions, placing the patient in a passive/reactive role. "I can't decrease how often I used the opioid medication because the others don't work as well." | Encourage a neutral approach to automatic thoughts as opposed to viewing these as internal mandates. Set specific, measurable, achievable, realistic, and time-limited goals with planned actions based on values, not emotions. |
| Cognitive Fusion | Rigid beliefs about the cause and effect of pain and pain management prevent the patient from engaging in health promotion behaviors. "I'll heal faster if I stay in bed because things that cause pain will harm me." | Find common ground by asking open-ended questions instead of criticizing a patient's understanding of pain. Within the limits of the patient's acceptance, establish shared goals that view pain as a mental construct. |

| Experimental Avoidance | Pain is worsened by the cycle of fear of pain, activity avoidance, decreased mobility and endurance, and impaired functioning. *"I can't try doing the things you said because it will cause more pain."* | Encourage shifting focus away from avoidance of negative experiences and moving toward positive experiences. Start with short-term goals that the patient feels they can accomplish. |

a Psychological barriers to postoperative recovery as described by Weinrib et al. in the approach by the Transitional Pain Service at the Toronto General Hospital.[36].
b Supportive care examples broadly reflect principles of CBT that may emphasize mindfulness, collaborative empiricism, goal setting, objective monitoring, and more specialized approaches such as Acceptability and Commitment Therapy (ACT).

- Pain severity from CPP or endometriosis
- Preoperative opioid use and whether chronic opioids will be tapered off or continued postoperatively
- Expectations for postoperative pain level and medication use
- Psychological comorbidities—specifically depression, anxiety, and pain catastrophizing

Severe side effects and poor analgesic responses may occur due to medication interactions or genetic differences in CYP enzyme activity. If this dyad occurs, we promptly change in an opioid metabolized in a different pathway, such as from tramadol to oxycodone, rather than dose or frequency escalation. Differentiating the use of opioids for treating postoperative pain versus chronic pain or nonpain symptoms (eg, poor sleep, anxiety) is critical to prevent inappropriate prescribing. Finally, multiple guidelines recommend against the use of long-acting opioids for the treatment of acute pain due to the risks of long-term dependence and difficulty in tapering.[32]

For patients who cannot use NSAIDs, have prior issues with poorly controlled perioperative pain, or have inadequate acute pain control with 40 MME per day, we often use either gabapentinoids and/or muscle relaxers. There are existing concerns about the concomitant use of these medications with opioids, but those risks must be weighed against the risks of further escalation of opioid therapy. The choice is guided by the presence of comorbid pain generators (eg, low back pain, pelvic floor myalgia) and, if responding to suboptimal pain control postoperatively, the character and location of pain (eg, nociceptive, neuropathic).

Few studies have evaluated the efficacy of nonpharmacological interventions for postoperative care in patients with CPP after hysterectomy. We find mindfulness-based stress reduction and gentle yoga to be particularly useful to increase mental and physical positive stimuli and to achieve functional outcomes. Outpatient regional nerve blocks or trigger point injections may target specific pain foci. Other strategies include ice packs, heating pads, nonrigid bracing devices, graduated exercise, and massage therapy.[32] Finally, clinicians are well-positioned to promote patient recovery through engaged and attentive care and encouragement of patients' support system to aid their care as well. These ideals are not always addressed in formal studies on chronic pain interventions but are likely major contributors to treatment success.

## SUMMARY

Hysterectomy remains an important treatment option for patients with CPP refractory to conservative therapy. Firm conclusions about its efficacy are impaired by the lack of a singular definition of CPP. Nonetheless, favorable outcomes have been reported for well-selected patients with only 5% to 26% of women reporting failure to achieve a significant or complete improvement in pain. Preoperative assessment should start with a comprehensive pain history to identify psychological comorbidities that predispose to chronic pain and to diagnose and treat COPCs as indicated. Patients are most likely to achieve relief from midline pelvic pain linked to the uterus by menstrual activity or tenderness on examination. Even for subgroups of patients with a high degree of central sensory sensitivity, hysterectomy for targeted symptoms has been shown to produce significant improvement in pain.

Surgical planning should address the need for the treatment of extrauterine pathology including deeply infiltrating endometriosis and ovarian removal. There is considerable benefit to ovarian conservation for young patients with modest increases in reoperation rate after hysterectomy. Beyond standard ERAS interventions, there are special postoperative considerations for patients with chronic pain including managing opioid use (preexisting and postoperative regimens), expanded use of non-opioid adjuvant medications, early treatment of complications or pain generators, and intentional communication strategies reflecting the biopsychosocial context for pain.

## CLINICS CARE POINTS

- A standardized history and examination for all patients with pelvic pain will aid in screening for COPCs (eg, BPS/IC) and in localizing specific sources of nonuterine pain (eg, levator ani myalgia).

- While psychological risk factors for centralized pain increase the risk of persistent or new pain after hysterectomy, these conditions should not preclude hysterectomy for patients with pain attributed to the uterus by history and/or examination.

- Success of hysterectomy is ultimately determined by the patient's goals and expectations, so we discuss and document that some symptoms (eg, dysmenorrhea) have a very high chance for resolution and others (eg, urinary urgency worsened during menses) are less predictable.

- In addition to multi-modal analgesia, patients with chronic pain benefit from supportive care that reinforces optimism and psychological flexibility.

## DISCLOSURE

Dr F. Tu has consulted for UroShape and Myovant. He conducts sponsored research with Eximis and Dot Laboratories. He receives royalties from Wolters Kluwer. Dr R. Cockrum has nothing to disclose.

## REFERENCES

1. Mathias SD, Kuppermann M, Liberman RF, et al. Chronic pelvic pain: prevalence, health-related quality of life, and economic correlates. Obstet Gynecol 1996; 87(3):321–7.
2. Merrill RM. Hysterectomy surveillance in the United States, 1997 through 2005. Med Sci Monit Int Med J Exp Clin Res 2008;14(1):CR24–31.
3. Brandsborg B, Nikolajsen L, Hansen CT, et al. Risk Factors for Chronic Pain after Hysterectomy: A Nationwide Questionnaire and Database Study. Anesthesiology 2007;106(5):1003–12.
4. Nicholas M, Vlaeyen JWS, Rief W, et al. The IASP classification of chronic pain for ICD-11: chronic primary pain. PAIN 2019;160(1):28–37.
5. Ghai V, Subramanian V, Jan H, et al. Evaluation of clinical practice guidelines (CPG) on the management of female chronic pelvic pain (CPP) using the AGREE II instrument. Int Urogynecol J 2021;32(11):2899–912.
6. American College of Obstetricians and Gynecologists. Chronic Pelvic Pain: Practice Bulletin 218. Obstet Gynecol 2020;135(3):e98–109.
7. Tu F, As-Sanie S. A modest proposal to investigate chronic uterine pain. BJOG Int J Obstet Gynaecol 2017;124(2):182–4.
8. Janda AM, As-Sanie S, Rajala B, et al. Fibromyalgia Survey Criteria Are Associated with Increased Postoperative Opioid Consumption in Women Undergoing Hysterectomy. Anesthesiology 2015;122(5):1103–11.
9. Brummett CM, Urquhart AG, Hassett AL, et al. Characteristics of fibromyalgia independently predict poorer long-term analgesic outcomes following total knee and hip arthroplasty. Arthritis Rheumatol Hoboken NJ 2015;67(5):1386–94.

10. Diatchenko L, Nackley AG, Slade GD, et al. Idiopathic pain disorders–pathways of vulnerability. Pain 2006;123(3):226–30.
11. Ghai V, Subramanian V, Jan H, et al. A systematic review on reported outcomes and outcome measures in female idiopathic chronic pelvic pain for the development of a core outcome set. BJOG Int J Obstet Gynaecol 2021;128(4):628–34.
12. Stovall TG, Ling FW, Crawford DA. Hysterectomy for Chronic Pelvic Pain of Presumed Uterine Etiology. Obstet Gynecol 1990;75(4):676–9.
13. Hillis SD, Marchbanks PA, Peterson HB. The Effectiveness of Hysterectomy for Chronic Pelvic Pain. Obstet Gynecol 1995;86(6):941–5.
14. Carlson KJ, Miller BA, Fowler FJJ. The Maine Women's Health Study: I. Outcomes of Hysterectomy. Obstet Gynecol 1994;83(4):556–65.
15. Tay SK, Bromwich N. Outcome of Hysterectomy for Pelvic Pain in Premenopausal Women. Aust N Z J Obstet Gynaecol 1998;38(1):72–6.
16. Hartmann KE, Ma C, Lamvu GM, et al. Quality of Life and Sexual Function After Hysterectomy in Women With Preoperative Pain and Depression. Obstet Gynecol 2004;104(4):701–9.
17. As-Sanie S, Till SR, Schrepf AD, et al. Incidence and predictors of persistent pelvic pain following hysterectomy in women with chronic pelvic pain. Am J Obstet Gynecol 2021;225(5):568.e1–11.
18. Meltzer-Brody S, Leserman J, Zolnoun D, et al. Trauma and posttraumatic stress disorder in women with chronic pelvic pain. Obstet Gynecol 2007;109(4):902–8.
19. Abu-Alnadi N, Frame B, Moore KJ, et al. Myofascial Pain in Hysterectomy Patients. J Minim Invasive Gynecol 2021;28(12):2067–72.
20. Chung MH, Huh CY. Comparison of treatments for pelvic congestion syndrome. Tohoku J Exp Med 2003;201(3):131–8.
21. Shakiba K, Bena JF, McGill KM, et al. Surgical treatment of endometriosis: a 7-year follow-up on the requirement for further surgery. Obstet Gynecol 2008; 111(6):1285–92.
22. Chung MK. Interstitial Cystitis in Persistent Posthysterectomy Chronic Pelvic Pain. JSLS 2004;8(4):329–33.
23. Lamvu G, Robinson B, Zolnoun D, et al. Vaginal Apex Resection: A Treatment Option for Vaginal Apex Pain. Obstet Gynecol 2004;104(6):1340–6.
24. Brandsborg B, Dueholm M, Nikolajsen L, et al. A Prospective Study of Risk Factors for Pain Persisting 4 Months After Hysterectomy. Clin J Pain 2009;25(4): 263–8.
25. Benlolo S, Hanlon JG, Shirreff L, et al. Predictors of Persistent Postsurgical Pain After Hysterectomy—A Prospective Cohort Study. J Minim Invasive Gynecol 2021;28(12):2036–46.e1.
26. Sangha R, Bossick A, Su WTK, et al. A Prospective Study of Patterns of Regret in the Year After Hysterectomy. J Patient-centered Res Rev 2020;7(4):329–36.
27. Parker WH, Feskanich D, Broder MS, et al. Long-term Mortality Associated with Oophorectomy versus Ovarian Conservation in the Nurses' Health Study. Obstet Gynecol 2013;121(4):709–16.
28. Richards L, Healey M, Cheng C, et al. Laparoscopic Oophorectomy to Treat Pelvic Pain Following Ovary-Sparing Hysterectomy: Factors Associated with Surgical Complications and Pain Persistence. J Minim Invasive Gynecol 2019;26(6): 1044–9.
29. Behera M, Vilos GA, Hollett-Caines J, et al. Laparoscopic findings, histopathologic evaluation, and clinical outcomes in women with chronic pelvic pain after hysterectomy and bilateral salpingo-oophorectomy. J Minim Invasive Gynecol 2006; 13(5):431–5.

30. Stone R, Carey E, Fader AN, et al. Enhanced Recovery and Surgical Optimization Protocol for Minimally Invasive Gynecologic Surgery: An AAGL White Paper. J Minim Invasive Gynecol 2021;28(2):179–203.

31. Keil DS, Schiff LD, Carey ET, et al. Predictors of Admission After the Implementation of an Enhanced Recovery After Surgery Pathway for Minimally Invasive Gynecologic Surgery. Anesth Analg 2019;129(3):776–83.

32. U.S. Department of Health and Human Services. Pain Management Best Practices Inter-Agency Task Force Rep Updates, Gaps, Inconsistencies, Recommendations. 2019. Available at: www.hhs.gov/opioids/prevention/pain-management-options/index.html. Accessed October 23, 2021.

33. As-Sanie S, Till SR, Mowers EL, et al. Opioid Prescribing Patterns, Patient Use, and Postoperative Pain After Benign Hysterectomy. Obstet Gynecol 2017;130(6):1261–8.

34. Till SR, Wahl HN, As-Sanie S. The role of nonpharmacologic therapies in management of chronic pelvic pain: what to do when surgery fails. Curr Opin Obstet Gynecol 2017;29(4):231–9.

35. Vandyken C, Hilton S. Physical Therapy in the Treatment of Central Pain Mechanisms for Female Sexual Pain. Sex Med Rev 2017;5(1):20–30.

36. Weinrib AZ, Azam MA, Birnie KA, et al. The psychology of chronic post-surgical pain: new frontiers in risk factor identification, prevention and management. Br J Pain 2017;11(4):169–77.

37. Wong M, Vogell A, Wright K, et al. Opioid use after laparoscopic hysterectomy: prescriptions, patient use, and a predictive calculator. Am J Obstet Gynecol 2019;220(3):259.e1–11.

38. Vilkins AL, Sahara M, Till S, et al. Effects of Shared Decision Making on Opioid Prescribing After Hysterectomy. Obstet Gynecol 2019;134(4):823–33.

# Role of Robotic Surgery in Benign Gynecology

Mireille D. Truong, MD*, Lauren N. Tholemeier, MD

## KEYWORDS

- Robotic surgery • Benign gynecology • Minimally invasive surgery
- Surgical simulation • Surgical innovation

## KEY POINTS

- Robotic surgery is a feasible and safe approach for various benign gynecologic procedures and has demonstrated superior perioperative outcomes compared with laparotomy for hysterectomy and myomectomy.
- The advancements in robotic surgical training have accelerated and shifted the paradigm for surgical training where simulation can decrease the learning curve for novice surgeons.
- Although cost is a commonly cited disadvantage of the robotic system, innovation and competition will likely drive down costs over time.

## BACKGROUND

### Historical Perspectives

Although the notion of robotic surgery dates to the 1960s, surgical robots were first used in the 1980s. The first Food and Drug Administration (FDA)-approved robotic device for intraabdominal surgery was introduced in 1994, followed by the first robotic surgery on a human in 1998. Tubal anastomosis was the first gynecologic procedure performed with robotic assistance (2000), followed by the first robotic hysterectomy in 2002.[1,2]

The initial impetus for development of a robotic system was due to the potential need for remote open surgery for military purposes. Through a collaboration of the Stanford Research Institute and the Defense Advanced Research Projects Agency, the first robotic system prototypes were developed,[3,4] which then led to the development of the AESOP surgical system, a predecessor to Da Vinci, which consisted of a voice-controlled camera arm for laparoscopy.[1] Next, ZEUS by Computer Motion was introduced, which included a camera arm, 2 robotic arms, and remote surgeon console. This was the first robotic device to be used for remote transatlantic surgery. After Computer Motion was acquired by Intuitive Surgical in 2003, the Da Vinci Surgical

Department of Obstetrics and Gynecology, Cedars-Sinai Medical Center, 444 South San Vicente Boulevard #1003, Los Angeles, CA 90048, USA
* Corresponding author. 8635 West Third Street, Suite 160W Los Angeles CA 90048.
E-mail address: Mireille.truong@cshs.org

Obstet Gynecol Clin N Am 49 (2022) 273–286
https://doi.org/10.1016/j.ogc.2022.02.009
0889-8545/22/© 2022 Elsevier Inc. All rights reserved.

System was developed. Since its FDA approval in 2005 for gynecologic surgery, robotic surgery has become a well-established approach for minimally invasive procedures in gynecology. Various robotic devices have since been developed ranging from multiport, to single port, to vaginal access platforms.[2,5]

### Technical Components and Features

Currently, the most widely used surgical robotic device is the DaVinci robotic system. This system provides several unique technologic advancements among endoscopic devices including 3-dimensional vision, higher magnification, tremor filtration, autonomous camera and energy instrument control, wrist articulation with 7° of freedom, telestration, and dual-console capabilities. These features can serve to improve ergonomics, visualization, dissection precision, and surgical training, while overcoming certain limitations of conventional laparoscopy such as counterintuitive hand movements, 2-dimensional visualization, limited degrees of instrument motion, and tremor amplification.[1,6]

### Indocyanine Green Fluorescence

Although not completely unique to the robotic system, the integration of indocyanine green (ICG) fluorescence technology with the Da Vinci robotic system has allowed ease of access and use of this technology across various surgical specialties for identification of anatomic and pathologic structures, including gynecologic surgery.[7]

Early pilot and observational studies have demonstrated feasibility, and its potential use for endometriosis surgery including intraoperative management, identification of lesions, and assessment of perfusion of bowel and ureter during deep infiltrating endometriosis resection.[8–10]

### Ergonomics

With the ability to sit and the increased dexterity of the robotic device, it has been suggested that robotic surgery confers better ergonomics compared to other modalities. Based on a survey by Santos-Carreras and colleagues of 49 surgeons with experience in all surgical approaches, there was less physical discomfort with robotic surgery compared with other modalities.[11] Although work-related musculoskeletal disorders (WMSD) have been reported for all surgical modalities, robot-assisted surgery has been related to lower rates of WMSDs.[12] A systematic review by Wee and colleagues reported that robotic surgery was associated with forearm, neck, and trapezius strain, but when compared with laparoscopy and open surgery, robotic surgery had lower muscular workload and improved ergonomics[13] This is an often-overlooked aspect of surgery but is an important consideration when evaluating the potential impact of long-term effects of ergonomics and WMSDs on surgeons' careers and the health care system.

## TRENDS IN GYNECOLOGIC ROBOTIC SURGERY

To better understand the role of robotics in benign gynecology, it is important to examine surgical trends since FDA approval in 2005. According to the American Association of Gynecologic Laparoscopists (AAGL) and the American College of Obstetrics and Gynecology (ACOG), hysterectomies should be performed minimally invasively when possible.[14,15] Despite the introduction of laparoscopic hysterectomy in 1989[16] and favorable outcomes data with minimally invasive approaches compared with laparotomy, in 2003 most hysterectomies were performed via laparotomy (66.1%), followed by vaginal (21.8%) and laparoscopic (11.8%).[17] Although the rate of laparoscopic hysterectomy has seen a gradual increase, robotic hysterectomy has had a more rapid adoption rate compared with conventional laparoscopic hysterectomy. A 2010 study of hospitals nationwide found that, within 5 years of FDA approval, robotic assistance was used for 10% of all hysterectomies. Among hospitals that offered robotic surgery, robotic assistance was used in nearly 25% of hysterectomies.[18] From 2005 to 2013, the percentage of all benign abdominal hysterectomies performed through laparotomy declined from 59% to 22%, as reported in the Premier Perspective database.[19] In 2012, there is an inflection point in trends where abdominal rates fall below minimally invasive hysterectomy rates, with 75% of hysterectomies were performed minimally invasively (MIS), with higher rates of robotic hysterectomy compared with other MIS approaches.[20] Several studies have demonstrated a parallel increase in robotic hysterectomy rates with a decrease in abdominal hysterectomies.[21–23] Similarly, according to a study by Dallas and colleagues, although laparotomy is still the most common method for performing myomectomy, since 2012 there is an increasing number of myomectomies performed minimally invasively, with a corresponding decrease in abdominal myomectomies.[24] Although many factors likely contribute to these trends, robotic surgery has certainly contributed to the decrease in laparotomy rates and its role continues to expand for benign gynecologic procedures.

## APPLICATIONS IN GYNECOLOGIC SURGERY: FEASIBILITY AND CLINICAL OUTCOMES

Robotic use for benign gynecologic procedures has demonstrated feasibility, safety, and equivalent clinical outcomes to conventional laparoscopy and better clinical outcomes compared with laparotomy.[25] The application of robotic approach has been described for various gynecologic procedures such as hysterectomy, myomectomy, sacrocolpopexy, endometriosis surgery, tubal reanastomosis, abdominal cerclage, isthmocele repair, and cesarean scar ectopic management. Although there are data to support feasibility for many of these applications, it is important to acknowledge the limited availability of high-quality studies and to take into consideration the challenges and limitations of surgical comparative studies. Biases and confounders such as surgeon volume, experience, and preference for surgical approach can affect the ability to adequately compare various surgical approaches.

### Hysterectomy

When compared with laparotomy, robotic hysterectomy has been shown to have lower blood loss, lower complication rates, and shorter length of stay.[26,27] In addition, robot-assisted hysterectomy has been demonstrated to be noninferior with respect to clinical outcomes when compared with conventional laparoscopic hysterectomy. A meta-analysis of randomized controlled trials (RCTs) comparing robot-assisted hysterectomy with conventional laparoscopic hysterectomy demonstrated no difference in rate of complications, operating time, length of hospital stay, blood loss, or conversion to laparotomy.[28] A retrospective cohort study of 8313 minimally invasive hysterectomies noted a lower overall complication rate in robotic group but no difference in major complication rate compared with other minimally invasive routes.[29] Initial studies where surgeons were early in their learning curve reported longer operative time for robot-assisted hysterectomy, but later studies suggest no difference in operative time.[30–32] Robot-assisted surgery is now a well-established approach for performing hysterectomy.

## Myomectomy

Although myomectomy is currently most often performed via laparotomy, robot-assisted surgery has been increasingly adopted as a feasible approach with improved perioperative outcomes. Several systematic reviews comparing robotic with open myomectomy found lower blood loss, lower complication rate, shorter hospital length of stay, and lower pain score but longer operative times.[33,34] Robot-assisted myomectomy has been shown to be noninferior to conventional laparoscopic myomectomy in terms of safety.[35] In a systematic review by Iavazzo and colleagues comparing robotic versus conventional laparoscopic myomectomy, there was no reported difference in complications, operative time, blood loss, or postoperative fertility. Notably, there were fewer conversions to open surgery in the robotic group, with conversion to open being 4 times more likely in the conventional laparoscopic group.[34] Similarly, Wang and colleagues found no difference in transfusion rates, complication rates, fibroid size, or operating time when comparing robot-assisted versus conventional laparoscopic myomectomy. They again found a lower risk of conversion to laparotomy and in this case a decrease in blood loss in the robotic group.[33] A 2021 systematic review on reproductive outcomes post-myomectomy reported no difference in pregnancy rates or outcomes with respect to surgical approach.[36] Although further data on reproductive outcomes are needed, robotic myomectomy should be considered as a minimally invasive option, given improved or similar perioperative outcomes compared with other modalities.

## Sacrocolpopexy

Given the unique features of the robotic device enhancing suturing and knot tying abilities, the robotic approach is particularly conducive for sacrocolpopexy . Robotic sacrocolpopexy has been shown to be feasible and safe with equivalent outcomes including anatomic cure rates and efficacy to the abdominal and laparoscopic approach.[37] A Cochrane review of RCTs comparing robot-assisted sacrocolpopexy with conventional laparoscopic sacrocolpopexy showed no difference in complications, blood transfusion, or conversion to laparotomy. This study did find a longer operative time in robot-assisted sacrocolpopexy, although this evidence was low quality.[38] Robotic sacrocolpopexy is therefore an effective minimally invasive option for apical prolapse repair.

## Endometriosis Surgery

Data evaluating the role of robotic surgery for the treatment of endometriosis are limited to retrospective studies with only one RCT comparing robotic with laparoscopic approach to date. However, based on current retrospective observational studies, the robotic platform has been demonstrated as a feasible, effective, safe, and advantageous tool for endometriosis surgery, particularly for complex endometriosis and resection of deep infiltrating endometriosis involving the bowels, bladder, and ureters.[39–41] Endometriosis resection involving the bowel has been successfully performed without complications or conversion to laparotomy.[42] A retrospective study comparing robotic and laparoscopic management of bladder endometriosis demonstrated similar rates of complications and recurrence.[43] The RCT (LAROSE trial) comparing robot-assisted versus conventional laparoscopic resection of endometriosis in 73 patientsfound no differences in operative time, blood loss, intraoperative or postoperative complications, or rates of conversion to laparotomy, with improvement in quality of life in both groups.[44] In addition, it has been reported that given improved visualization from 3D vision and higher magnification with the robotic camera, there is better detection of endometriosis lesions compared with conventional laparoscopic camera. One study demonstrated 80% detection of endometriosis biopsy-confirmed lesions with robotic compared with 56.8% with laparoscopic approach (P < .001).[45,46] Robotic surgery for management of endometriosis is feasible and may provide certain benefits, but prospective studies are warranted to further evaluate outcomes and better define its role for the treatment of endometriosis.

### Cesarean Scar Ectopic and Isthmocele Repair

An isthmocele is a defect in the uterine myometrium resulting from a previous cesarean delivery for which laparoscopic, vaginal, hysteroscopic, and robotic approaches for repair have been reported. Although there is a paucity of data for all modalities, robotic surgery is an emerging approach and has been demonstrated to be feasible for the removal of cesarean scar pregnancies and isthmocele repair, which can be performed concurrently.[47,48] One case report describes treatment of cesarean scar ectopic pregnancy with parenteral methotrexate followed by robot-assisted removal of residual pregnancy tissue with repair of the defect, leading to a subsequent intrauterine pregnancy.[49] Another patient underwent successful robot-assisted removal of a cesarean scar ectopic after failed methotrexate therapy.[50] In a case series of 5 patients, medical treatment with lidocaine and methotrexate injection was followed by surgery at least 2 months later. Hysteroscopy was used to identify the ectopic and remove as much pregnancy tissue as possible using the cold resectoscope loop followed by robot-assisted laparoscopic removal of residual tissue and isthmocele repair.[51] Although feasibility and safety have been demonstrated, more evidence is needed to clarify the role of the robotic approach for cesarean scar ectopic and isthmocele repair and to compare outcomes with other modalities.

### Tubal anastomosis

As previously mentioned, tubal anastomosis was the first application of robotics in gynecologic surgery. This procedure can be challenging with the laparoscopic and open approach, given the need for microsuturing. The robotic device is therefore particularly applicable for this procedure, as it can overcome the challenges related to suturing due to improved visualization, increased magnification, decreased tremor, and the use of articulating instruments. A single institution analysis of robotic tubal anastomosis reported decreasing operative time with experience (140.7 ± 27.0 minutes for the first 11 case vs 60.0 ± 9.1 minutes last 26 cases of the study period). In this study, the pregnancy rate was 59% and tubal patency rate was 81%, which is consistent with other surgical approaches' outcomes.[52] A systematic review in 2017 on tubal anastomosis showed no difference in outcomes between microscopic laparotomy, laparoscopic, and robotic techniques.[53] Therefore, robotic technique is an acceptable noninferior approach for tubal anastomosis.

### Cerclage

Although the first reported robot-assisted laparoscopic cerclage was performed in 2007, the studies for robotic cerclage are limited to case reports and series with only one retrospective comparative study. In this study by Smith and colleagues, the robotic and open approaches were compared. Robot-assisted cerclage was found to have similar obstetric outcomes but associated with decreased blood loss and shorter hospitalizations compared with laparotomy.[54] In a case series, cost of robotic cerclage was reported to be equivalent to laparotomy.[55] Robot-assisted cerclage is feasible and may be superior to laparotomy. However, the robotic application for transabdominal cerclage needs to be further evaluated.

## OTHER SURGICAL CONSIDERATIONS
### Complex Cases

Higher complexity cases can be approached with various minimally invasive techniques based on procedure type, patient characteristics, and surgeon experience. In some instances, the use of robotics may confer certain advantages, such as autonomy when limited or no assistance is available, with improved or similar perioperative outcomes compared with other surgical approaches. A study by Advincula and Reynolds was one of the first feasibility studies to suggest a potential role for robotics in overcoming technical limitations of conventional laparoscopy for hysterectomy cases with obliterated anterior cul-de-sac.[56] In a retrospective cohort study, the difference in operative time for high-volume surgeons treating "complex" patients with robot-assisted hysterectomy versus laparoscopic hysterectomy was 21 minutes faster ($P < .05$). Complex patients were defined as having a body mass index of 45 kg/m$^2$ or greater, uterine weight of 700 g or more, or past diagnosis of adhesions. The study concluded that operative time with robotic surgery may be shorter for patients with complex disease in the hands of an experienced surgeon, with no difference in complications.[57] Another retrospective study comparing surgical approaches with myomectomy noted that myoma weight in the robotic and abdominal group was much higher than laparoscopic group (263, 220, 96 g, respectively, $P = .002$). The robotic group also had a higher total number of myomas compared with laparoscopic, suggesting that robot assistance allows for completion of more complex cases.[58] In another retrospective study by Lim and colleagues, robot-assisted hysterectomy cases were of higher complexity (older patients, higher rate of adhesive disease, larger uteri) but with lower complications and length of stay and similar conversion rate compared with the other approaches.[19] The surgical robot should be considered as an additional tool for complex gynecologic procedures.

### Combined Multispecialty Cases

The robotic system can also be used as a tool to facilitate combined cases with multiple surgical specialties; this is most applicable in cases where surgeons in a multidisciplinary team are proficient with the robotic device and all use the robotic approach for their portion of a procedure. In a case report, Moawad and colleagues describe a case of deep infiltrating endometriosis requiring collaboration between urology, gynecology, and colorectal surgery. The robotic system was used by all 3 specialties and allowed for a smooth transition between each portion of the procedure.[59] The feasibility of multispecialty robotic cases has been demonstrated, although further studies are needed.[60]

### Learning Curve and Operative Time

There has been conflicting evidence regarding operative time for robotic surgery compared with other surgical approaches. Although the robotic device has been used for gynecology for over 20 years, many studies reflect the early learning curve for robotic gynecologic procedures compared with other modalities that have preceded robotic surgery. There is evidence that with increasing volume, operative time is expected to improve. The learning curve for robotic hysterectomy has been reported to range between 20 and 100 cases, with decreased operative time and complication rates once the learning plateau has been reached. Bell and colleagues described operative time for the first 20 cases to be an average of 124 minutes followed by 94 minutes in the second 20 cases. Complications were highest in the first

20 at 15%, compared with 5% for the remaining groups, but this did not reach statistical significance, and this suggests that competency can be reached after 20 cases.[61] In a study of "high-volume" surgeons who have performed at least 50 cases, the operative time for robot-assisted hysterectomy was shorter than laparoscopic hysterectomy, 147 minutes versus 174 minutes. However, this study was underpowered to detect a significant difference.[32] High-volume surgeons performing robot-assisted hysterectomy showed a decrease in operative time after 75 cases despite an increase in uterine weight.[21] Among surgeons who had performed at least 60 of their respective type of hysterectomy, rate of complications and length of stay were lower in robotic group compared with other approaches.[19]

Set up and docking the robotic system have often been described as time consuming steps that lead to prolonged operative time. However, with an experienced team, docking time can be significantly reduced and have a minimal impact on operative time. In the first 90 robot-assisted hysterectomies performed at their institution, Kho and colleagues achieved a mean docking time of 2.95 minutes (standard deviation 1.77 minutes).[62]

## TRAINING AND SIMULATION

The advancements in robotic surgical training have accelerated and shifted the paradigm for surgical training. The detached surgeon console and the lack of haptics, although sometimes considered limitations, have proved to be advantageous in the development of robotic surgical training tools such as virtual and augmented reality simulation, dual consoles, integrated digital capture, machine learning, and artificial intelligence. Multiple virtual reality robotic simulators have been developed incorporating discreet skills and, procedural and team training.[63] Turner and Kim describe mapping the robotic hysterectomy learning curve with simulator metrics to individualize training for residents. They noted objective improvement in use of the robot, such as fewer collisions and better efficiency of movement, with additional simulation practice.[64] The dual console, unique to the robotic system, allows surgeons to cooperate not only with other surgeons but also with trainees and therefore facilitates intraoperative teaching with real-time feedback.[65]

Animate and inanimate laboratories have been used for surgical training but with limited effectiveness for robotic training due to cost and accessibility. Robotic surgery lends itself to digital and virtual training tools, which can improve access and is conducive for both synchronous and asynchronous learning with ability of real-time feedback. Integration of video capture and artificial intelligence technology such as Crowd-Sourced Assessment of Technical Skills (C-SATS), Proximie, and Orpheus will further expand training capabilities, as these tools have the potential to provide learners with remote intraoperative proctoring or coaching and objective digital analytics, assessments, and feedback. Although face and content validities have been established for virtual reality simulators,[66] cost can still be a challenge. In addition, the integration of these tools into robotic surgical curricula, the transferability of skills to the operating room, and the impact on clinical outcomes still need to be further evaluated.

## CREDENTIALING

Credentialing is not currently standardized and is generally determined by individual institutions. Suggested guidelines for credentialing processes have been provided by the AAGL and ACOG, which include simulation, proctoring, case review, annual cases minimums, and progression from "basic" to "advanced" procedures.[67,68] One hospital outlined their robust credentialing process that involves a stepwise approach including dry laboratory, proctored cases, peer review, and annual case minimums.[69]

## CHALLENGES IN ROBOTIC GYNECOLOGIC SURGERY
### Access to Minimally Invasive Gynecologic Surgery

There are significant disparities in patient access to minimally invasive surgery. Older age, black race, Hispanic ethnicity, and smaller hospital size are associated with lower likelihood of undergoing minimally invasive hysterectomy.[70] These disparities extend to, and are in some cases worse for, robotic hysterectomy. In a cross-sectional study using the 2012 to 2014 National Inpatient Sample, patients were more likely to undergo robotic hysterectomy if the hospital is large, for profit, or a teaching institution. In contrast, patients were less likely to undergo robotic hysterectomy if they are rural, African American, uninsured, or publicly insured. In this study, findings were adjusted for surgical indications, including fibroids; therefore, racial disparities occurred independently of type of pathology.[71] Another single institution study found that women were less likely to undergo robot-assisted hysterectomy if they were African American, enrolled in Medicaid, or in the lowest income quartile.[72] Factors contributing to the disparities in access to minimally invasive gynecologic surgery are multifold, and further evaluation of these disparities are beyond the scope of this article. However, it is important to note that although location and cost of robotic systems may be contributing to these disparities, the robotic device offers an additional minimally invasive tool that can help decrease the rate of laparotomy and bridge the gap between disparities in gynecologic surgical techniques. Access to minimally invasive gynecologic surgery, including robotics, is an important consideration, as new robotic devices are implemented in the health care system and in the development of future robotic devices.

### Cost

Although there are limited retrospective data on costs for robotic gynecologic procedures, cost of robotic surgery remains an area of criticism. Cost evaluation is complex and can be challenging to evaluate comparatively due to varying factors affecting cost such as surgery technique, instrument selection, surgeon experience, and consideration for indirect versus direct costs; this may account for the heterogeneity of cost calculations among studies evaluating cost for robotic surgery. When compared with other minimally invasive approaches, studies have reported increased cost associated with robotic gynecologic procedures such as hysterectomy, myomectomy, and sacrocolpopexy.[73] However, when the robotic device is considered a preexisting investment, similar costs were noted between robotic and laparoscopic hysterectomy (Lonnerfors 2015).[74] In addition, when compared with laparotomy, the robotic approach is often less expensive for hysterectomy and for sacrocolpopexy.[75,76]

Cost can be addressed at the surgeon, hospital, and global level. The robotic device is still considered a relatively new endoscopic technology, especially for gynecologic procedures other than hysterectomy, and therefore, with increasing surgeon experience, there can be an expected decrease in operative time and complications over time, which can help decrease cost.[22] Improvements in training and utilization of simulation to shorten learning curve may also improve cost. With surgeon education, cost transparency, and appropriate selection of instrumentation, costs have been shown to decrease.[77] At the hospital level, cost can be mitigated by incorporating a multispecialty robotic program that can help maximize utilization and volume, and by negotiating cost plans such as leasing options. The introduction of competing robotic systems can further drive down costs.[78]

## FUTURE DIRECTIONS

Since its first application in gynecologic surgery over 25 years ago, robotic surgery has been established as a feasible and safe approach for various gynecologic procedures with superior or equivalent outcomes to laparotomy and noninferior outcomes compared with conventional laparoscopy. Although not the sole factor, the addition of robotic surgery as a minimally invasive technique has had an impact in decreasing rates of laparotomy in gynecologic surgery. Significant focus has been placed on robot-assisted hysterectomy, given that hysterectomy is the most common benign gynecologic procedure. However, robotics plays an important role in other gynecologic surgeries such as myomectomy, where most of these procedures are still being performed via laparotomy.

Although on occasion, it has previously beendescribed as a technological gimmick, the robotic system represents a step in the evolution of endoscopy. Robotic surgery expands on fundamental components of endoscopy such as a camera and minimal incision sizes with unique features that enhance surgical dexterity, precision, visualization, and training. These features can facilitate management of complex cases such as large masses, extensive adhesive disease, advanced endometriosis, cases requiring extensive suturing, surgery in obese patients and combined surgical cases. Although remote surgery was an initial intention of the robotic system, it has not yet been widely adopted as such due to challenges with latency. Recent advances in technology and the current pandemic have led to an increased interest in remote training, proctoring, and coaching.

In addition to prioritizing patient safety and outcomes, surgeon well-being is an important consideration. With improved ergonomics and less physical strain, adoption of robotics may improve surgeon longevity and minimize work-related injuries.

Robotic surgery for benign gynecologic surgery continues to expand and provides several unique technological advantages. As with any technology, there must be space and balance between innovation and evidence to allow for the robotic device to evolve. With the development of the next generation of robotic devices, limitations such as size of the device, cost, access, and training should be addressed while maintaining current benefits, patient safety, high-quality care, and good clinical outcomes.

## CLINICS CARE POINTS

- Robotic surgery is a feasible and safe approach for various benign gynecologic procedures.
- Equivalent perioperative outcomes between robotic and other minimally invasive approaches have been demonstrated for hysterectomy, myomectomy, sacrocolpopexy, and endometriosis surgery.
- Robot-assisted surgery has demonstrated superior perioperative outcomes compared with laparotomy for hysterectomy and myomectomy.
- The role for robotic approach is to be further evaluated for tubal anastomosis, cerclage, and management of cesarean scar ectopic and isthmocele repair.
- The advancements in robotic surgical training have accelerated and shifted the paradigm for surgical training where simulation can decrease the learning curve for novice surgeons.
- Robotic surgery confers better ergonomics compared with other modalities, potentially minimizing work-related musculoskeletal disorders.

**DISCLOSURE**

The authors of this review have no relevant financial interests to disclose. This review was not funded.

## REFERENCES

1. George EI, Brand TC, LaPorta A, et al. Origins of robotic surgery: from skepticism to standard of care. JSLS 2018;22(4). e2018.00039.
2. Mendivil A, Holloway RW, Boggess JF. Emergence of robotic assisted surgery in gynecologic oncology: American perspective. Gynecol Oncol 2009;114(2 Suppl):S24–31.
3. Visco AG, Advincula AP. Robotic gynecologic surgery. Obstet Gynecol 2008; 112(6):1369–84.
4. Advincula AP, Wang K. Evolving role and current state of robotics in minimally invasive gynecologic surgery. J Minim Invasive Gynecol 2009;16(3):291–301.
5. Peters BS, Armijo PR, Krause C, et al. Review of emerging surgical robotic technology. Surg Endosc 2018;32(4):1636–55.
6. Cho JE, Nezhat FR. Robotics and gynecologic oncology: review of the literature. J Minim Invasive Gynecol 2009;16(6):669–81.
7. Lee SY, Koo YJ, Lee DH. Classification of endometriosis. Yeungnam Univ J Med 2021;38(1):10–8.
8. Bar-Shavit Y, Jaillet L, Chauvet P, et al. Use of indocyanine green in endometriosis surgery. Fertil Steril 2018;109(6):1136–7.
9. Raimondo D, Borghese G, Mabrouk M, et al. Use of indocyanine green for intraoperative perfusion assessment in women with ureteral endometriosis: a preliminary study. J Minim Invasive Gynecol 2021;28(1):42–9.
10. Cosentino F, Vizzielli G, Turco LC, et al. Near-infrared imaging with indocyanine green for detection of endometriosis lesions (Gre-Endo Trial): a pilot study. J Minim Invasive Gynecol 2018;25(7):1249–54.
11. Santos-Carreras L, Hagen M, Gassert R, et al. Survey on surgical instrument handle design: ergonomics and acceptance. Surg Innov 2012;19(1):50–9.
12. Catanzarite T, Tan-Kim J, Whitcomb EL, et al. Ergonomics in surgery: a review. Female Pelvic Med Reconstr Surg 2018;24(1):1–12.
13. Wee IJY, Kuo LJ, Ngu JC. A systematic review of the true benefit of robotic surgery: Ergonomics. Int J Med Robot 2020;16(4):e2113.
14. AAGL Advancing Minimally Invasive Gynecology Worldwide. AAGL position statement: route of hysterectomy to treat benign uterine disease. J Minim Invasive Gynecol 2011;18(1):1–3.
15. Robot-assisted surgery for noncancerous gynecologic conditions: ACOG COMMITTEE OPINION SUMMARY, Number 810. Obstet Gynecol 2020;136(3):640–1.
16. Reich H, Decaprio J, McGlynn F. Laparoscopic hysterectomy. J Gynecol Surg 1989;5:213–7.
17. Wu JM, Wechter ME, Geller EJ, et al. Hysterectomy rates in the United States, 2003. Obstet Gynecol 2007;110(5):1091–5.
18. Wright JD, Ananth CV, Lewin SN, et al. Robotically assisted vs laparoscopic hysterectomy among women with benign gynecologic disease. JAMA 2013;309(7): 689–98.
19. Lim PC, Crane JT, English EJ, et al. Multicenter analysis comparing robotic, open, laparoscopic, and vaginal hysterectomies performed by high-volume surgeons for benign indications. Int J Gynaecol Obstet 2016;133(3):359–64.

20. Pitter MC, Simmonds C, Seshadri-Kreaden U, et al. The impact of different surgical modalities for hysterectomy on satisfaction and patient reported outcomes. Interact J Med Res 2014;3(3):e11.
21. Carbonnel M, Moawad GN, Tarazi MM, et al. Robotic hysterectomy for benign indications: what have we learned from a decade? JSLS 2021;25(1). e2020.00091.
22. AlAshqar A, Goktepe ME, Kilic GS, et al. Predictors of the cost of hysterectomy for benign indications. J Gynecol Obstet Hum Reprod 2021;50(2):101936.
23. Smorgick N, Patzkowsky KE, Hoffman MR, et al. The increasing use of robot-assisted approach for hysterectomy results in decreasing rates of abdominal hysterectomy and traditional laparoscopic hysterectomy. Arch Gynecol Obstet 2014; 289(1):101–5.
24. Dallas K, Molina A, Siedhoff M, et al. Myomectomy Trends in a population-based cohort from 2005-2018. J Minim Invasive Gynecol 2021;28(Supplement 11):S125.
25. Truong M, Kim JH, Scheib S, et al. Advantages of robotics in benign gynecologic surgery. Curr Opin Obstet Gynecol 2016;28(4):304–10.
26. Matthews CA, Reid N, Ramakrishnan V, et al. Evaluation of the introduction of robotic technology on route of hysterectomy and complications in the first year of use. Am J Obstet Gynecol 2010;203:499.e1-5.
27. Landeen LB, Bell MC, Hubert HB, et al. Clinical and cost comparisons for hysterectomy via abdominal, standard laparoscopic, vaginal and robot-assisted approaches. S D Med 2011;64:197–9, 201, 203 passim.
28. Albright BB, Witte T, Tofte AN, et al. Robotic versus laparoscopic hysterectomy for benign disease: a systematic review and meta-analysis of randomized trials. J Minim Invasive Gynecol 2016;23(1):18–27.
29. Swenson CW, Kamdar NS, Harris JA, et al. Comparison of robotic and other minimally invasive routes of hysterectomy for benign indications. Am J Obstet Gynecol 2016;215(5):650.e1-8.
30. Paraiso MR, Ridgeway B, Park AJ, et al. A randomized trial comparing conventional and robotically assisted total laparoscopic hysterectomy. Am J Obstet Gynecol 2013;208:368.e1–7.
31. Sarlos D, Kots L, Stevanovic B, et al. Robotic compared with conventional laparoscopic hysterectomy. A randomized controlled trial. Obstet Gynecol 2012;120: 604–11.
32. Lonnefors C, Reynisson P, Persson J. A randomized trial comparing vaginal and laparoscopic hysterectomy vs robotic-assisted hysterectomy. J Minim Invasive Gynecol 2015;22:78–86.
33. Wang T, Tang H, Xie Z, et al. Robotic-assisted vs. laparoscopic and abdominal myomectomy for treatment of uterine fibroids: a meta-analysis. Minim Invasive Ther Allied Technol 2018;27(5):249–64.
34. Iavazzo C, Mamais I, Gkegkes ID. Robotic assisted vs laparoscopic and/or open myomectomy: systematic review and meta-analysis of the clinical evidence. Arch Gynecol Obstet 2016;294(1):5–17.
35. Gkegkes ID, Iatrakis G, Iavazzo PE, et al. Robotic management of fibroids: discussion of use, criteria and advantages. Acta Med (Hradec Kralove) 2020; 63(2):63–6.
36. Orlando M, Kollikonda S, Hackett L, et al. Non-hysteroscopic myomectomy and fertility outcomes: a systematic review. J Minim Invasive Gynecol 2021;28(3): 598–618.e1.
37. Ko KJ, Lee KS. Robotic sacrocolpopexy for treatment of apical compartment prolapse. Int Neurourol J 2020;24(2):97–110.

38. Lawrie TA, Liu H, Lu D, et al. Robot-assisted surgery in gynaecology. Cochrane Database Syst Rev 2019;4(4):CD011422.
39. Nezhat C, Hajhosseini B, King LP. Robotic-assisted laparoscopic treatment of bowel, bladder, and ureteral endometriosis. JSLS 2011;15(3):387–92.
40. Liu C, Perisic D, Samadi D, et al. Robotic-assisted laparoscopic partial bladder resection for the treatment of infiltrating endometriosis. J Minim Invasive Gynecol 2008;15(6):745–8.
41. Hur C, Falcone T. Robotic treatment of bowel endometriosis. Best Pract Res Clin Obstet Gynaecol 2021;71:129–43.
42. Kang J, Kim J. The role of robotic surgery for endometriosis. Gyne Robot Surg 2020;1(2):36–49.
43. Carpentier M, Merlot B, Bot Robin V, et al. Partial cystectomy for bladder endometriosis: robotic assisted laparoscopy versus standard laparoscopy. Gynecol Obstet Fertil 2016;44:315–21.
44. Soto E, Luu TH, Liu X, et al. Laparoscopy vs. robotic surgery for endometriosis (LAROSE): a multicenter, randomized, controlled trial. Fertil Steril 2017;107(4):996–1002.e3.
45. Dulemba JF, Pelzel C, Hubert HB. Retrospective analysis of robot-assisted versus standard laparoscopy in the treatment of pelvic pain indicative of endometriosis. J Robot Surg 2013;7(2):163–9.
46. Mosbrucker C, Somani A, Dulemba J. Visualization of endometriosis: comparative study of 3-dimensional robotic and 2-dimensional laparoscopic endoscopes. J Robot Surg 2018;12(1):59–66.
47. Schmitt A, Crochet P, Agostini A. Robotic-assisted laparoscopic treatment of residual ectopic pregnancy in a previous cesarean section scar: a case report. J Minim Invasive Gynecol 2017;24(3):342–3.
48. Yoon R, Sasaki K, Miller CE. Laparoscopic excision of cesarean scar pregnancy with scar revision. J Minim Invasive Gynecol 2021;28(4):746–7.
49. Siedhoff MT, Schiff LD, Moulder JK, et al. Robotic-assisted laparoscopic removal of cesarean scar ectopic and hysterotomy revision. Am J Obstet Gynecol 2015;212(5):681.e1–6814.
50. Kashi PK, Dengler KL, Welch EK, et al. A stepwise approach to robotic assisted excision of a cesarean scar pregnancy. Obstet Gynecol Sci 2021;64(3):329–31.
51. Hoffmann E, Vahanian S, Martinelli VT, et al. Combined medical and minimally invasive robotic surgical approach to the treatment and repair of cesarean scar pregnancies. JSLS 2021;25(3). e2021.00039.
52. Ghomi A, Nolan W, Rodgers B. Robotic-assisted laparoscopic tubal anastomosis: Single institution analysis. Int J Med Robot 2020;16(6):1–5.
53. van Seeters JAH, Chua SJ, Mol BWJ, et al. Tubal anastomosis after previous sterilization: a systematic review. Hum Reprod Update 2017;23(3):358–70.
54. Smith RB, Brink J, Hu C, et al. Robotic transabdominal cerclage vs Laparotomy: a comparison of obstetric and surgical outcomes. J Minim Invasive Gynecol 2020;27(5):1095–102.
55. Lee R, Biats D, Mancuso M. Robotic transabdominal cerclage: a case series illustrating costs. J Robot Surg 2018;12(2):361–4.
56. Advincula AP, Reynolds RK. The use of robot-assisted laparoscopic hysterectomy in the patient with a scarred or obliterated anterior cul-de-sac. JSLS 2005;9(3):287–91.
57. Herrinton LJ, Raine-Bennett T, Liu L, et al. Outcomes of robotic hysterectomy for treatment of benign conditions: influence of patient complexity. Perm J 2020;24:19.035.

58. Barakat EE, Bedaiwy MA, Zimberg S, et al. Robotic-assisted, laparoscopic, and abdominal myomectomy: a comparison of surgical outcomes. Obstet Gynecol 2011;117(2 Pt 1):256–66.

59. Moawad GN, Tyan P, Abi Khalil ED, et al. Multidisciplinary Resection of Deeply Infiltrative Endometriosis. J Minim Invasive Gynecol 2018;25(3):389–90.

60. Piccoli M, Esposito S, Pecchini F, et al. Full robotic multivisceral resections: the Modena experience and literature review. Updates Surg 2021;73(3):1177–87.

61. Bell MC, Torgerson JL, Kreaden U. The first 100 da Vinci hysterectomies: an analysis of the learning curve for a single surgeon. S D Med 2009;62(3):91–5.

62. Kho RM, Hilger WS, Hentz JG, et al. Robotic hysterectomy: technique and initial outcomes [published correction appears in Am J Obstet Gynecol. 2007 Sep;197(3):332]. Am J Obstet Gynecol 2007;197(1):113.e1–1134.

63. Julian D, Tanaka A, Mattingly P, et al. A comparative analysis and guide to virtual reality robotic surgical simulators. Int J Med Robot 2018;14:10.

64. Turner TB, Kim KH. Mapping the robotic hysterectomy learning curve and re-establishing surgical training metrics. J Gynecol Oncol 2021;32(4):e58.

65. Azadi S, Green IC, Arnold A, et al. Robotic surgery: the impact of simulation and other innovative platforms on performance and training. J Minim Invasive Gynecol 2021;28(3):490–5.

66. Culligan P, Gurshumov E, Lewis C, et al. Predictive validity of a training protocol using a robotic surgery simulator. Female Pelvic Med Reconstr Surg 2014;20(1):48–51.

67. Guidelines for privileging for robotic-assisted gynecologic laparoscopy. AAGL Advancing Minimally Invasive Gynecology Worldwide. J Minim Invasive Gynecol 2014;21:157–67.

68. American College of Obstetricians and Gynecologists' Committee on Gynecologic Practice, The Society of Gynecologic Surgeons. Robot-Assisted Surgery for Noncancerous Gynecologic Conditions: ACOG COMMITTEE OPINION, Number 810. Obstet Gynecol 2020;136(3):e22–30.

69. Rardin CR. The debate over robotics in benign gynecology. Am J Obstet Gynecol 2014;210(5):418–22.

70. Mehta A, Xu T, Hutfless S, et al. Patient, surgeon, and hospital disparities associated with benign hysterectomy approach and perioperative complications. Am J Obstet Gynecol 2017;216(5):497.e1–10.

71. Smith AJB, AlAshqar A, Chaves KF, et al. Association of demographic, clinical, and hospital-related factors with use of robotic hysterectomy for benign indications: A national database study. Int J Med Robot 2020;16(4):e2107.

72. Price JT, Zimmerman LD, Koelper NC, et al. Social determinants of access to minimally invasive hysterectomy: reevaluating the relationship between race and route of hysterectomy for benign disease. Am J Obstet Gynecol 2017;217(5):572.e1–10.

73. Lim CS, Griffith KC, Travieso J, et al. To robot or not to robot: the use of robotics in benign gynecologic surgery. Clin Obstet Gynecol 2020;63(2):327–36.

74. Lonnerfors C, Reynisson P, Persson J. A randomized trial comparing vaginal and laparoscopic hysterectomy vs robot-assisted hysterectomy. J Minim Invasive Gynecol 2015;22:78–86.

75. Kaaki B, Lewis E, Takallapally S, et al. Direct cost of hysterectomy: comparison of robotic versus other routes. J Robot Surg 2020;14(2):305–10.

76. Oliver JL, Kim JH. Robotic sacrocolpopexy-is it the treatment of choice for advanced apical pelvic organ prolapse? Curr Urol Rep 2017;18(9):66.
77. Misal M, Delara R, Wasson MN. Cost-effective minimally invasive gynecologic surgery: emphasizing surgical efficiency. Curr Opin Obstet Gynecol 2020; 32(4):243–7.
78. Wu CZ, Klebanoff JS, Tyan P, et al. Review of strategies and factors to maximize cost-effectiveness of robotic hysterectomies and myomectomies in benign gynecological disease. J Robot Surg 2019;13(5):635–42.

# Laparoscopic Abdominal Cerclage

Shabnam Gupta, MD[a,b],*, Jon Ivar Einarsson, MD, PhD, MPH[a,b]

## KEYWORDS

- Laparoscopic abdominal cerclage • Cervical insufficiency
- Minimally invasive gynecology

## KEY POINTS

- Laparoscopic abdominal cerclage is a highly effective, well-tolerated surgical treatment of patients with refractory cervical insufficiency or anatomic limitations to vaginal cerclage.
- Transabdominal cerclage is preferred for patients with cervical insufficiency and a prior failed vaginal cerclage, given improved birth outcomes compared with repeat transvaginal cerclage.
- Suggested benefits of abdominal cerclage compared with vaginal cerclage include a more proximal placement at the level of the internal os, greater mechanical support to the cervix, decreased risk of caudal suture migration as pregnancy progresses, and possible reduced risk of ascending intrauterine infections due to the absence of foreign body material in the vagina.
- Neonatal survival rates more than 96% and mean gestational age of 37 weeks at delivery have been observed in subsequent pregnancies with laparoscopic abdominal cerclage in place.

## INTRODUCTION

Preterm birth is a significant cause of infant morbidity and mortality. A well-established cause of preterm birth is cervical insufficiency, which occurs in up to 8% of women with a history of miscarriage and approximately 1% of all pregnancies.[1] Recommended treatment of patients with cervical insufficiency includes a cerclage placement or procedure in which a stitch is tied around the cervix. Cerclages function by providing structural support to the cervix and keeping it artificially closed throughout pregnancy. Cerclages can be placed transvaginally or transabdominally. In this article, we will discuss transabdominal cerclages with emphasis placed on the indications, surgical technique, and clinical outcomes associated with a minimally invasive approach.

[a] Brigham & Women's Hospital, Harvard Medical School, 75 Francis Street, CWN 3rd Floor, MIGS Office, Boston, MA 02115, USA; [b] Division of Minimally Invasive Gynecology, Harvard Medical School, 75 Francis Street, CWN 3rd Floor, MIGS Office, Boston, MA 02115, USA
* Corresponding author.
E-mail address: sgupta44@bwh.harvard.edu
Twitter: @ShabnamGuptaMD (S.G.)

Obstet Gynecol Clin N Am 49 (2022) 287–297
https://doi.org/10.1016/j.ogc.2022.02.010
0889-8545/22/© 2022 Elsevier Inc. All rights reserved.

obgyn.theclinics.com

### Cervical Insufficiency

Cervical insufficiency is defined as an inability of the uterine cervix to maintain a pregnancy in the second-trimester, without signs of labor, clinical contractions, or both.[2] This often follows painless cervical dilation or cervical shortening. While the clinical presentation can vary, this condition often presents around 16 to 18 weeks of gestation with subsequent preterm or previable delivery.

Structural weakness of the cervix can be a result of cervical trauma (prior operative vaginal deliveries, surgery of the cervix or uterus including loop electrosurgical excision or conization, mechanical dilation during pregnancy terminations) or congenital abnormalities (collagen disorders such as Ehlers–Danlos syndrome, Mullerian anomalies, in utero diethylstilbestrol exposure).[3] Second-trimester births and fetal losses can also be caused by infection or decidual inflammation, bleeding at the decidua-placenta interface, or overdistension of the uterus. These each result in biochemical changes in the cervix leading to shortening and/or dilation with subsequent preterm delivery.

In select cases, a cerclage can be placed to prevent second-trimester loss or subsequent preterm birth in a pregnancy affected by painless cervical dilation or very short cervix. This is termed a rescue cerclage. Alternatively, a cerclage can be placed prophylactically or before conception in women with a history of previous preterm deliveries or fetal losses due to cervical insufficiency.

### Discussion

#### History of cerclages

Transvaginal cerclage placement was first described by Shirodkar and McDonald in the 1950s.[4,5] Traditionally, cerclages have been placed with nonabsorbable sutures via a vaginal approach. In the McDonald procedure, a simple, purse-string suture is inserted at the cervicovaginal junction. In the Shirodkar procedure, the stitch is placed higher up on the cervix, requiring the dissection of the vesicocervical mucosa to expose tissue closer to the level of the internal cervical os. The suture is then placed, and the mucosa is closed back over the secured knot. Surgeon preference typically guides treatment approach, as neither surgical technique has demonstrated superior outcomes.[6,7]

In 1965, Benson and Durfee proposed a transabdominal approach to cerclage placement at the cervicoisthmic junction.[8] This approach differed from the historically performed Shirodkar and McDonald techniques which place the cerclage more distally at the intersection of the cervix and vaginal fornix (**Fig. 1**). The laparoscopic approach to transabdominal cerclage was first reported in 1998 and has been gaining increased popularity since this time (**Fig. 2**).[9]

## WHEN TO CONSIDER TRANSABDOMINAL CERCLAGE

Transabdominal cervicoisthmic cerclage was initially suggested for women with a history of cervical insufficiency and anatomy that precluded a transvaginal cerclage (history of trachelectomy, inadequate vaginal access). Over the past 50 years, abdominal cerclage indications have been expanded to also include women with refractory cervical insufficiency.[10]

Women who have experienced a second-trimester fetal loss or preterm birth despite an appropriately timed and placed transvaginal cerclage are considered to have refractory cervical insufficiency and should be offered an abdominal cerclage (**Fig. 3**). It is important to rule out other causes of second-trimester loss including large fibroids or Mullerian anomalies with a thorough history and imaging studies as needed.

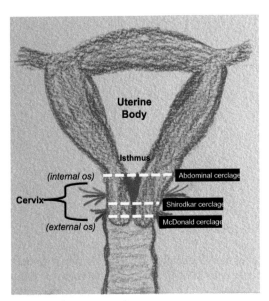

**Fig. 1.** Anatomic placement of various cerclage types.

Recent evidence suggests that an abdominal cerclage improves neonatal outcomes compared with repeat vaginal cerclage in patients with one prior failed vaginal cerclage.[11] Providers should individualize counseling and adhere to principles of beneficence and nonmaleficence to help each patient reach their unique reproductive health goals.

A recent 2020 landmark randomized controlled trial of abdominal versus vaginal cerclage (the MAVRIC trial or Multicentre Abdominal vs Vaginal Randomized Intervention of Cerclage) has provided substantial validation for the belief that an abdominal approach is a preferred approach for patients with cervical insufficiency and a prior failed vaginal cerclage given improved birth outcomes and superior reduction in risk of early preterm birth and fetal loss in women with previous failed vaginal cerclage compared with repeat transvaginal placement.[12] This study evaluated 111 women with a single prior failed vaginal cerclage (fetal loss or preterm birth between 14 and 28 weeks of gestation). Patients were randomized to either an open abdominal cerclage or repeat vaginal cerclage placement. Results of this trial found that preterm birth

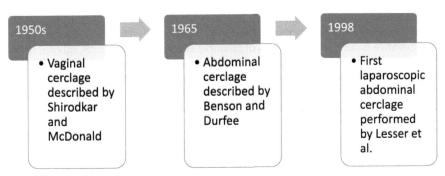

**Fig. 2.** Historical timeline of cerclage use.

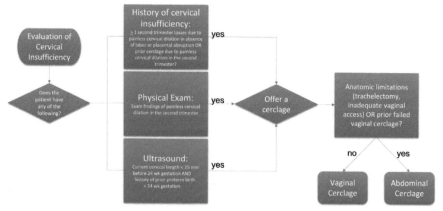

**Fig. 3.** Cerclage decision tree.

before 32 weeks of gestation occurred in only 8% of women randomized to an abdominal cerclage, compared with 38% of women randomized to a repeat vaginal cerclage ($P = .008$).

Contraindications to transabdominal cerclage are similar to those for transvaginal cerclage. Clinical scenarios in which cerclages are unlikely to reduce the risk of preterm birth or improve fetal outcomes include fetal anomalies incompatible with life, intrauterine infections, active uterine bleeding, active labor, preterm rupture of membranes, and fetal demise. A relative contraindication includes the presence of prolapsed fetal membranes through the external cervical os. In these cases, the potential risk of iatrogenic rupture of membranes may exceed 50%.[2,6]

## ADVANTAGES OF A LAPAROSCOPIC, MINIMALLY INVASIVE APPROACH

The advantage of the abdominal approach compared with the vaginal approach is the ability to place the suture at or slightly above the level of the internal os, providing greater mechanical support to the cervix. There is also decreased risk of caudal suture migration as pregnancy progresses and the uterus enlarges.[13] Additionally, an abdominal cerclage avoids the prolonged presence of a foreign body within the vagina, which may reduce the potential for ascending infections and resulting preterm labor or premature rupture of membranes.

Transabdominal cerclage has been underutilized in the past due to the need for cesarean section, risk of intraoperative blood loss at the uterine vessels, and historically, the need for a laparotomy with associated morbidity (risks of poor postoperative pain control, overnight hospital admission, and delayed return to normal activities). Laparoscopy has many benefits over laparotomy, including smaller incisions with faster postoperative healing, reduced risks of postoperative wound infections, quicker return to baseline function, less blood loss, and ability to undergo outpatient surgery.[14] While the cesarean section is still required for delivery, increased surgeon experience and more widespread use of minimally invasive surgery has encouraged more physicians to offer laparoscopic abdominal cerclage to patients with the aforementioned indications.

Moawad and colleagues noted in a systematic review of laparoscopic abdominal cerclage that neonatal outcomes were similar compared with laparotomy. In this review, 1844 women who underwent laparoscopically versus open abdominal cerclage were found to have no significant difference in neonatal survival rates (90% for laparoscopic and 91% for open cerclage, $P = .8$).[15] Of note, after excluding first trimester losses from the analysis, women who underwent laparoscopic abdominal cerclage had significantly greater neonatal survival rates (97% vs 90%, $P < .01$). First trimester losses are unlikely to be related to cervical insufficiency or cerclage placement and can, therefore, be appropriately excluded.

### Timing of Laparoscopic Abdominal Cerclage

Laparoscopic cerclages are ideally placed prior to conception (termed an interval cerclage) for multiple reasons. The nonpregnant uterus is smaller in size and can accommodate a uterine manipulator. These factors give the surgeon better visualization of anatomy for proper cerclage placement. Surgeons face additional challenges including increased paracervical vasculature, blood supply, and tissue softness with a gravid uterus.[13] Preconception abdominal cerclage placement is associated with lower rates of repeat spontaneous pregnancy loss and preterm labor, and less surgical and pregnancy-related morbidity compared with postconception placement.[16] Studies have shown that preconception cerclage placement does not impact fertility.[17]

Optimal timing for laparoscopic abdominal cerclage placement in pregnancy is the late first trimester or early second trimester (8–12 weeks). This time period reduces the risk of miscarriage associated with earlier gestation, enables time for exclusion of major anomalies from aneuploidy screening and ultrasound studies, and ensures that the uterus is not too large, which can make cerclage placement more technically challenging. More advanced pregnancies can be offered abdominal cerclage placement after appropriately counseling, depending on the clinical picture and surgeon experience. Postconception cerclage placement confers a small risk of fetal loss, with estimated rates of 1.2% in laparoscopic cases and 3% of open cases.[12]

### SURGICAL TECHNIQUE

Here we will describe our surgical approach to laparoscopic abdominal cerclage placement in a nonpregnant patient. No prophylactic antibiotics are administered before incision. Laparoscopic abdominal cerclage placement is performed under general anesthesia with the patient in the dorsal lithotomy position. A catheter is placed in the bladder to keep it decompressed throughout the procedure. Port placement is guided by surgeon preference. We prefer to use 4 ports: a 10-mm scope at the umbilicus, two 5-mm ports in the bilateral lower quadrants, and a fourth ipsilateral port in the left upper quadrant. In nonpregnant women, a uterine manipulator is placed to assist with the traction and delineation of planes for proper angulation and placement of the suture needle. No manipulator is placed in a gravid uterus, although a sponge stick could be considered.

The procedure starts with the dissection of the vesicouterine peritoneum to expose the uterine arteries anteriorly and move the bladder slightly caudad (**Fig. 4**).

Next, a 5-mm Mersilene polyester tape with blunt-tip needles on either side is used for cerclage placement. This is the same tape commonly used for transvaginal cerclages. The blunt-tip needles are straightened out before insertion using heavy-duty needle holders (**Fig. 5**). We find that the needles are unnecessarily long for laparoscopic cerclages, thus grasping the needle closer to the tip can help with needle management.

The posterior broad ligament is not opened before needle insertion, as opening this area can add the unnecessary risk of underlying vessel injury. Direct insertion of the needle simplifies the procedure and has not led to any complications thus far. The ureter is identified, and its course is followed distally (**Fig. 6**).

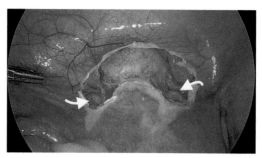

**Fig. 4.** Dissection of the anterior vesicouterine peritoneum. The uterine arteries are indicated by white arrows.

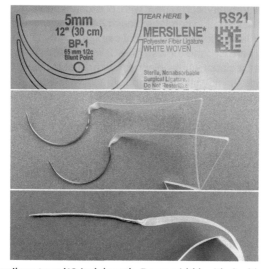

**Fig. 5.** A single Mersilene tape (12-inch length, 5-mm width) with double-armed blunt point needles is used for laparoscopic abdominal cerclage. The curved needles are straightened to allow for insertion through laparoscopic trocars and to aid in needle handling.

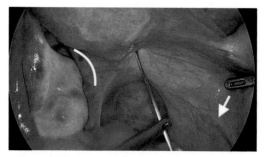

**Fig. 6.** Placement of the first needle on the right. The uterine artery is indicated with a red arrow, the ureter with a white arrow, and the site of anticipated needle insertion on the left is shown with a blue dot. The curved white line highlights the lateral border of the cervix.

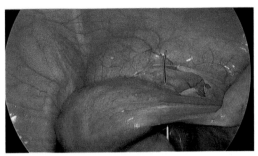

**Fig. 7.** Twisting the uterus with the uterine manipulator (*left hand*) enables the surgeon to better visualize the correct exit point and direct the needle placement (*right hand*).

Our preference is to insert the suture posteriorly at the level of the internal cervical os, just above the insertion of the uterosacral ligaments. It can be helpful to think of the uterus and cervix as an hourglass, with the level of the internal os as the narrowest point of the hourglass. The suture is carefully passed in the space between the uterine vessels and cervical stroma. The uterine artery (identified by its pulsation) should be lateral to the placement of the needle, and the uterosacral ligament should be below. The use of blunt needles is advantageous because it enables the surgeon to direct the needle more medially to avoid uterine vessels, and then adjust placement more laterally if the resistance of the cervix is encountered. Proper placement of suture follows a low resistance path. We find it helpful to twist the uterus with the uterine manipulator in one hand, while placing and directing the needle path in tandem with the other hand (**Fig. 7**). Once the needles are passed bilaterally, they are cut off the Mersilene tape and removed through the ports.

The 2 free ends of the Mersilene tape are then pulled anteriorly to ensure that the suture is tightened and flush with the posterior cervix. The tape is then secured using intracorporeal knot tying. It is important to ensure that the first and second knots are tied down snuggly and flat against the anterior cervix. We find it helpful to have the assistant hold down the first knot with a grasper, so that it doesn't slip while the second knot is tied (**Fig. 8**). Our approach is to secure 6 square knots.

Once the knots have been secured, the tape is trimmed and secured to the lower uterine segment with a 2.0 silk suture to prevent a theoretic risk of erosion into the bladder (**Fig. 9**).

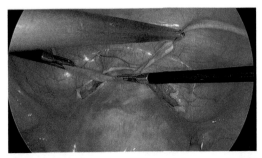

**Fig. 8.** An assistant grasps the knot to prevent slippage to secure the first square knot flush with the anterior cervix.

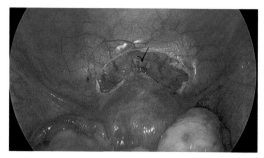

**Fig. 9.** The free ends of the tied Mersilene tape have been secured with silk suture.

Next, the overlying vesicouterine peritoneum is closed with 2 to 0 Monocryl suture using intracorporal knot tying (**Fig. 10**).

Finally, all instruments are removed from the abdomen and pelvis, and port sites are closed.

Significant bleeding or severe complications are rarely encountered.[11] In the case of oozing from the uterine vein, this will often resolve once the Mersilene stitch is tied down. Persistent bleeding even after securing the cerclage may require additional placement of a simple figure of 8 stitches (Monocryl or Vicryl) at the posterior insertion of the tape to obtain hemostasis.

## POSTOPERATIVE COURSE

Due to the advantages of a minimally invasive surgical approach, patients can undergo laparoscopic abdominal cerclage as an outpatient procedure, without the need for overnight hospital admission. Pain is controlled adequately with nonnarcotic medications including ibuprofen and acetaminophen. Postoperative restrictions include performing activities as tolerated, with recommendations for 2 weeks of pelvic rest. Most patients experience a return to baseline function within 1 to 2 weeks. Patients may begin attempts at conception 2 months after laparoscopic abdominal cerclage placement. We recommend that they receive obstetric care as high-risk patients.

## WHEN TO REMOVE AN ABDOMINAL CERCLAGE

Abdominal cerclages can be removed at the time of cesarean delivery if the patient has completed her childbearing. If the patient is still considering future childbearing, the cerclage can be left in place for future pregnancies. In the event of a miscarriage,

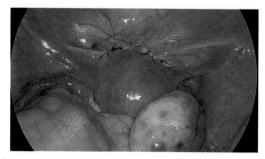

**Fig. 10.** The anterior vesicouterine peritoneum has been closed.

a dilation and curettage procedure can be performed with the abdominal cerclage in place up to 18 weeks of gestation.[18] For more advanced gestational ages, hysterotomy may be necessary if the patient desires to keep the cerclage, or laparoscopic removal of the cerclage can be performed to allow for the vaginal passage of the fetus.

## CLINICAL OUTCOMES

As with all surgical procedures, technical skill and surgeon experience are important factors for successful patient outcomes. At the Brigham & Women's Hospital in Boston, we have been performing abdominal cerclages for more than 20 years and were one of the first centers in the United States to offer a laparoscopic, minimally invasive approach to placement. Since 2007, we have performed more than 150 laparoscopic abdominal cerclage placements. Most of these patients had at least one prior second-trimester loss (many of them had multiple losses), with many having also failed a transvaginal cerclage (**Table 1**). In an analysis of 169 of these cases, the neonatal survival rate was 96.9% in the 98 pregnancies that followed and extended beyond the first trimester, and the mean gestational age at delivery was 37.0 weeks (first trimester losses are typically excluded from the denominator because they are unlikely to be the result of cervical insufficiency).[11]

**Table 1**
**Laparoscopic abdominal cerclage in 169 patients at the Brigham & Women's Hospital in Boston, Massachusetts**

| Parameters | Values |
|---|---|
| Patient Characteristics (n = 169) | |
|   Mean Age (y)[a] | 34.9 ± 4.5 |
|   History | |
|     First Trimester Loss | 77 (45.6%) |
|     Second-Trimester Loss | 125 (45.6%) |
|     Third Trimester Loss | 6 (3.6%) |
|     Previous Transvaginal Cerclage | 112 (66.3%) |
|     Cervical Surgery or Injury | 104 (61.5%) |
| Procedural Outcomes (n = 169) | |
|   Mean Operative Time (min)[a] | |
|     All Cases | 61 ± 36 |
|     No Additional Procedures | 49 ± 25 |
|   Mean Estimated Blood Loss (mL)[a] | |
|     All Cases | 23 ± 20 |
|     No Additional Procedures | 17 ± 11 |
|   Complications | 2 (1.2%) |
|   Same-day Discharge | 163 (96.4%) |
| Obstetric Outcomes (n = 98) | |
|   Neonatal Survival Rate[b] | 96 (96.9%) |
|   Mean Gestational Age (wk)[a] | 37.0 ± 1.3 |
|   Mean Birth Weight (g)[a] | 2963 ± 459 |

[a] Mean ± standard deviation.
[b] Neonates surviving until hospital discharge.

## SUMMARY

Laparoscopic abdominal cerclage is a minimally invasive, highly effective surgical treatment of patients with refractory cervical insufficiency or anatomic limitations to vaginal cerclage placement. The laparoscopic abdominal technique has demonstrated similar or improved neonatal survival rates compared with the more invasive, historically performed open approach.

## CLINICS CARE POINTS

- Cervical insufficiency is a well-established cause of infant morbidity and mortality
- Cervical cerclage placement is the recommended treatment of women with cervical insufficiency
- Cerclages can be placed transvaginally or transabdominally
- Women with anatomic limitations to vaginal cerclage placement or prior failed vaginal cerclages should be offered transabdominal cerclage placement
- Abdominal cerclage requires cesarean delivery
- Abdominal cerclage is the preferred approach for patients with cervical insufficiency and a prior failed vaginal cerclage gave improved birth outcomes compared with repeat transvaginal placement
- Benefits of abdominal cerclages compared with vaginal cerclages include a more proximal placement at the level of the internal os, greater mechanical support to the cervix, decreased risk of caudal suture migration with the progression of pregnancy, and possible reduced risk of ascending intrauterine infections due to the absence of foreign body material in the vagina
- Laparoscopic abdominal cerclage is the preferred approach compared with laparotomy
- Benefits of laparoscopic approach includes smaller incisions, faster postoperative healing, reduced risk of postoperative wound infections, quicker return to baseline function, less blood loss, and ability to undergo outpatient surgery
- Laparoscopic cerclages are ideally placed before conception but can be placed up to the early second trimester of pregnancy
- Patients with abdominal cerclage should receive obstetric care as high-risk patients
- Abdominal cerclages can be removed during cesarean delivery if the patient has completed childbearing, otherwise it can be left in place for pregnancies
- Dilation and curettage can be performed through abdominal cerclage placement up to 18 weeks of gestation
- Neonatal survival rates more than 96% and mean gestational age of 37 weeks at delivery have been observed in subsequent pregnancies with laparoscopic abdominal cerclage in place
- Laparoscopic abdominal cerclage is a highly effective, well-tolerated surgical treatment of refractory cervical insufficiency or anatomic limitations to vaginal cerclage placement

## DISCLOSURE

S. Gupta has nothing to disclose; J.I. Einarsson is a consultant for Olympus, Hologic and Arthrex.

## REFERENCES

1. Thakur M, Mahajan K. Cervical incompetence. StatPearls; 2021. Available at: https://www.ncbi.nlm.nih.gov/books/NBK525954/.

2. American College of Obstetricians and Gynecologists. ACOG Practice Bulletin No. 142: Cerclage for the management of cervical insufficiency. Obstet Gynecol 2014;123:372–9.
3. Leduc L, Wasserstrum N. Successful treatment with the Smith-Hodge pessary of cervical incompetence due to defective connective tissue in Ehlers-Danlos syndrome. Am J Perinatol 1992;9(1):25.
4. Shirodkar V. A new method of operative treatment of habitual abortions in the second trimester of pregnancy. Antiseptic 1955;52:299–300.
5. McDonald IA. Suture of the cervix for inevitable miscarriage. J Obstet Gynaecol Br Emp 1957;64(3):346–50.
6. Harger JH. Cerclage and cervical insufficiency: an evidence-based analysis. Obstet Gynecol 2002;100:1313.
7. Berghella V, Szychowski JM, Owen J, et al. Suture type and ultrasound-indicated cerclage efficacy. Vaginal ultrasound trial consortium. J Matern Fetal Neonatal Med 2012;25:2287–90.
8. Benson RC, Durfee RB. Transabdominal cervicouterine cerclage during pregnancy for the treatment of cervical incompetency. Obstet Gynecol 1965;25: 145–55.
9. Lesser KB, Childers JM, Surwit EA. Obstet Gynecol. 1998;91:855–6.
10. Witt MU, Joy SD, Clark J, et al. Cervicoisthmic cerclage: transabdominal vs transvaginal approach. Am J Obstet Gynecol 2009;201(1):105.e1–1054.
11. Clark N, Einarsson J. Laparoscopic abdominal cerclage: a highly effective option for refractory cervical insufficiency. Fertil Steril 2020. https://doi.org/10.1016/j.fertnstert.2020.02.007.
12. Shennan A, Chandiramani M, Bennett P, et al. MAVRIC: a multicentre randomised controlled trial of transabdominal versus transvaginal cervical cerclage. Am J Obstet Gynecol 2020;222(3):261.e1–9.
13. Ari S, Akdemir A, Sendag F. Transabdominal cervical cerclage. Non-obstetric surgery during pregnancy. Springer; 2019. p. 355–60.
14. Medeiros LR, Stein AT, Fachel J, et al. Laparoscopy versus laparotomy for benign ovarian tumor: a systematic review and meta-analysis. Int J Gynecol Cancer 2008;18(3):387–99.
15. Moawad GN, Tyan P, Bracke T, et al. Systematic review of transabdominal cerclage placed via laparoscopy for the prevention of preterm birth. J Minim Invasive Gynecol 2018;25:277–86.
16. Dawood F, Farquharson RG. Transabdominal cerclage: preconceptual versus first trimester insertion. Eur J Obstet Gynecol Reprod Biol 2016;199:27–31.
17. Vousden NJ, Carter J, Seed PT, et al. What is the impact of preconception abdominal cerclage on fertility: evidence from a randomized controlled trial. Acta Obstet Gynecol Scand 2017;96(5):543–6.
18. Chandiramani M, Chappell L, Radford S, et al. Successful pregnancy following mid-trimester evacuation through a transabdominal cervical cerclage. BMJ Case Rep 2011. https://doi.org/10.1136/bcr.02.2011.3841. bcr0220113841.

# Emerging Treatment Options for Fibroids

Briana L. Baxter, MD[a],*, Hye-Chun Hur, MD, MPH[a], Richard S. Guido, MD[b]

## KEYWORDS

- Fibroids • Abnormal uterine bleeding • Uterine-sparing • Fertility enabling

## KEY POINTS

- Uterine fibroids are common benign tumors that can significantly alter the quality of life of patients.
- The options for minimally invasive and nonsurgical treatments have significantly increased in the last decade.
- Clinicians must become familiar with these new technologies to adequately counsel their patients.

## BACKGROUND

Leiomyomas or fibroids are extremely common in reproductive aged patients. They are monoclonal tumors that develop from the uterine myometrium and are almost always benign. Fibroids are dependent on estrogen and progesterone, and as such, most fibroids shrink after menopause.[1] Fibroids are commonly classified by their topographic location in the uterus. Generally, fibroids are termed subserosal (located within the serosal layer of the uterus), intramural (located within the contractile smooth muscle of the uterus), or submucosal (located within the endometrial lining). However, many fibroids have a hybrid presentation with both a subserosal and intramural component, an intramural and submucosal component, or a transmural presentation with subserosal, intramural, and submucosal components. Therefore, to establish a universal and more detailed classification system, the International Federation of Gynecology and Obstetrics (FIGO) (**Fig. 1**) created the now widely used eight-type FIGO Leiomyoma Subclassification System (2011).[2] Submucosal fibroids are classified as Type 0 (pedunculated intracavitary), Type 1 (less than 50% intramural), and Type 2 (more than 50% intramural). Intramural fibroids are classified as Type 3 to Type 6. Type 3 fibroids contact the endometrium, and Types 5 to 6 are either less than 50%

[a] Division of Gynecologic Specialty Surgery, Department of Obstetrics & Gynecology, Columbia University Irving Medical Center, New York, NY 10032, USA; [b] Department of Obstetrics, Gynecology and Reproductive Sciences, Magee-Womens Hospital of University of Pittsburgh Medical Center, Pittsburgh, PA 15213, USA
* Corresponding author.
*E-mail address:* blb2167@cumc.columbia.edu

Obstet Gynecol Clin N Am 49 (2022) 299–314
https://doi.org/10.1016/j.ogc.2022.03.001

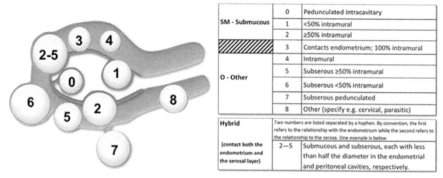

| | 0 | Pedunculated intracavitary |
|---|---|---|
| SM - Submucous | 1 | <50% intramural |
| | 2 | ≥50% intramural |
| | 3 | Contacts endometrium; 100% intramural |
| | 4 | Intramural |
| O - Other | 5 | Subserous ≥50% intramural |
| | 6 | Subserous <50% intramural |
| | 7 | Subserous pedunculated |
| | 8 | Other (specify e.g. cervical, parasitic) |
| Hybrid | | Two numbers are listed separated by a hyphen. By convention, the first refers to the relationship with the endometrium while the second refers to the relationship to the serosa. One example is below |
| (contact both the endometrium and the serosal layer) | 2—5 | Submucous and subserous, each with less than half the diameter in the endometrial and peritoneal cavities, respectively. |

Fig. 1. Leiomyoma Subclassification System. (*Adapted from* Munro MG, Critchley HO, Broder MS, Fraser IS; FIGO Working Group on Menstrual Disorders. FIGO classification system (PALM-COEIN) for causes of abnormal uterine bleeding in nongravid women of reproductive age. Int J Gynaecol Obstet. 2011;113(1):3-13. https://doi.org/10.1016/j.ijgo.2010.11.011; with permission.)

or more than 50% subserosal. Pedunculated subserosal fibroids are classified as Type 7, and fibroids that are cervical, parasitic, etc., are classified as Type 8. The system also allows for classification of "hybrid leiomyomas" or fibroids that impact multiple layers as a range of stages. For example, a fibroid with a less than 50% submucosal component and less than 50% subserosal components is termed Type 2 to 5.[2,3]

Clinically, management of fibroids can be challenging, especially if childbearing is not complete. Patients may present with abnormal uterine bleeding, pressure or bulk symptoms, infertility, and/or pain, whereas some may have no symptoms at all. Additionally, beyond physical symptoms, fibroids are associated with a significant burden on a patient's emotional and psychosocial health.[4] Fibroids are a public health concern, with annual fibroid-related treatment costs estimated to be as high as $34.4 billion in the United States.[5] Treatment options can be classified as medical, procedural, or surgical. Despite advances in both medical and procedural treatments, symptomatic fibroids remain the most common indication for hysterectomy.[6] However, many patients desire uterine preservation for a variety of reasons, including fertility preservation, maintenance of body integrity, cultural factors, and/or personal preferences. Notably, hysterectomy, even when performed with ovarian conservation, can shorten the time to menopause by 2 to 4 years, which may lead to an increased risk of cardiovascular disease.[7] Thus, when considering fibroid treatment options, important considerations include severity of symptoms, health status, age, surgical risks, family planning goals, and the patient's desire for uterine preservation.

The emerging treatments we present here are nonresective and thus do not allow for definitive tissue diagnosis. Leiomyosarcoma (LMS) is a rare, aggressive, malignant tumor identified in 0.36 per 100,000 women-years. It is difficult to distinguish LMS from a benign leiomyoma preoperatively, and unfortunately there is no standard preoperative assessment.[8] Dynamic MRI and lactate dehydrogenase isoenzyme testing have been suggested to identify LMS preoperatively; however, the evidence is based on limited clinical studies.[9] There are no data supporting biopsy of leiomyomas. Additionally, owing to the low prevalence of this disease, positive predictive values are low. Clearly additional research and techniques are required to better risk-stratify individuals for their risk of this rare diagnosis. However, the prevalence of LMS in presumed leiomyomas is low; in a systematic review by the Agency for Healthcare Research and Quality

(AHRQ) in 2017, the estimated risk of an unexpected LMS is between 1 and 13 per 10,000 surgeries performed for symptomatic fibroids.[9]

Available fibroid treatments include medical (hormonal & nonhormonal), procedural (uterine artery embolization [UAE]), MRI-guided ultrasound ablation (high-intensity focused ultrasound [HIFU]), and surgical options (myomectomy, hysterectomy, and ablative techniques).[10,11] This article will focus on emerging therapies that allow for uterine-sparing, fertility-enabling treatment (**Table 1**).

## MEDICAL THERAPIES

Medical therapies for fibroids are usually directed at managing heavy menstrual bleeding (HMB) or bulk symptoms. Comparative data between medical treatments are limited; thus, fibroid management is often guided by patient factors such as medical comorbidities and safety, desire for fertility, tolerability, ancillary benefits (ie, contraceptive), and cost.

### Heavy Menstrual Bleeding

Medical therapies for HMB include hormonal and nonhormonal options. Nonhormonal medical options include nonsteroidal anti-inflammatory drugs (NSAIDs) and tranexamic acid, both of which are usually taken during menses. In contrast, hormonal options are typically taken throughout the cycle. Hormonal options include combined estrogen–progesterone contraceptives, progestin-only contraceptives, (Gonadotropin releasing hormone (GnRH) analogs, and selective progesterone receptor modulators (**Table 2**).

NSAIDs have been studied for treatment of HMB due to fibroids owing to the presumed impact they may play on elevated prostaglandin levels seen in patients with fibroids. However, a Cochrane review published in 2019 found that although NSAIDs reduced HMB compared with placebo, they were significantly less effective than tranexamic acid or the levonorgestrel intrauterine device (LNG-IUD).[12] Tranexamic acid is a synthetic antifibrinolytic drug that is available in both oral and intravenous formulations and can reduce bleeding up to 40%.[13] It is typically administered orally, initiated with onset of menses, and used for up to 5 days during the menstrual cycle.[6]

| Table 1 Treatment options for fibroids | | |
|---|---|---|
| **Medical** | **Procedural (Nonresective Treatments)** | **Surgical (Fibroid Resection)** |
| Nonhormonal medications (nonsteroidal anti-inflammatory drugs, tranexamic acid) | Uterine artery embolization (UAE) | Myomectomy (hysteroscopic, laparoscopic/robotic, open) |
| Combined oral contraceptives (COCs) | High-intensity focused ultrasound (HIFU) | Hysterectomy (vaginal, laparoscopic/robotic, open) |
| Progestin-only options (pills, injection, implants, IUD) | | Radiofrequency ablation (RFA)[a] |
| GnRH analogs (Lupron, Oriahnn, Myfembree) | | |
| Selective progesterone receptor modulators (SPRMs) | | |

[a] Radiofrequency ablation techniques are *nonresective surgical* procedure.

**Table 2**
**Medical management options for fibroids**

| Heavy Menstrual Bleeding | Bulk Symptoms |
|---|---|
| Nonhormonal medications (NSAIDS, tranexamic acid) | GnRH analogs (Lupron, Oriahnn, Myfembree) |
| Combined oral contraceptives (COCs) | Selective progesterone receptor modulators (SPRMs) |
| Progestin-only contraceptives (pills, injection, implants, IUD) | |
| GnRH analogs (Lupron, Oriahnn, Myfembree) | |
| Selective progesterone receptor modulators (SPRMs) | |

Although there is little evidence supporting the use of combined estrogen–progesterone contraceptives for treatment of HMB due to fibroids, it is typically used as a first-line medical treatment for fibroid-related bleeding. Combined estrogen–progesterone contraceptives are available in many forms including pills, patch, and ring. The choice of formulation can be left to the patient's preference and compliance patterns. In addition to medical treatment of HMB, combined oral contraceptives offer other health benefits including contraception, reduction of uterine and ovarian cancer, ovarian cyst suppression, and potential treatment of acne.[11,13–15] Clinicians who prescribe combined contraceptive therapy for the treatment of menorrhagia due to fibroids should be aware of the various contraindications to their use.[16]

For patients with contraindications to estrogen therapy or for those who choose to avoid estrogen-containing methods, progesterone-only therapies are available. Progesterone-only treatments are available in many formulations including the pill, implant, injection, and IUD, with varying degrees of efficacy in the reduction of HMB. Among the progesterone-only options, the LNG-IUD is associated with the greatest reduction in blood loss compared with placebo or alternative hormonal medical treatments.[10,17] Currently, the American College of Obstetricians and Gynecologists (ACOG) supports the use of the 52-mg LNG-IUD for the treatment of abnormal uterine bleeding due to fibroids. It is important to note that rates of IUD expulsion are higher in patients with fibroids (11%) than in patients without fibroids (0%–3%). Additionally, the risk for expulsion seems to be higher for patients with fibroids distorting the cavity.[11,14]

GnRH analogs are either agonists (leuprolide) or antagonists (elagolix and relugolix) that inhibit the hypothalamic–pituitary–ovarian axis, resulting in a decrease in estrogen levels.[10,11] GnRH agonists have been used for the treatment of fibroids for many years and are associated with a reduction in fibroid size, total uterine volume, and menstrual bleeding. Leuprolide is typically dosed at one- or 3-month intervals and is administered as a depot injection. GnRH suppression typically occurs after 7 to 14 days and is preceded by an initial "flare" where a transient increase in Luteinizing hormone (LH) and Follice Stimulating Hormone (FSH) can cause a temporary worsening of HMB.[6,14] Because GnRH agonists work by inducing hypogonadism, use is often limited by hypoestrogenic adverse effects such as menopausal symptoms, unfavorable changes in lipid profile, and/or decrease in bone density. GnRH agonists are often used preoperatively as a surgical adjunct to improve anemia and decrease total uterine size or as a bridge to natural menopause for perimenopausal patients. The Food and Drug Administration (FDA)–approved labeling for fibroids states that leuprolide is approved for concomitant use with iron therapy for preoperative hematologic improvement of patients with anemia caused by fibroids for whom 3 months of hormonal suppression is deemed necessary. It is not approved with norethindrone acetate add-back specifically for the preoperative hematologic improvement prior to surgery. Treatment is typically limited to 6 months but can be used for up to 1 year if used with add-back therapy or concomitant use with low-dose estrogen and/or progestin.[6,11]

GnRH antagonists also decrease estrogen levels by inhibiting LH and FSH and similarly significantly improve fibroid-related HMB. However, GnRH antagonists are available in oral preparations and are conveniently formulated with low-dose add-back to limit hypoestrogenic side effects.[18] Oral GnRH antagonists, elagolix and relugolix, in combination with estradiol and norethindrone acetate have recently been FDA-approved for the treatment of fibroid-related HMB for up to 24 months of use. Elagolix is formulated with add-back therapy in the twice daily administered Oriahnn and is associated with significant reduction in HMB from baseline.[19] Alternatively, relugolix combination therapy (Myfembree) is administered once daily and is also associated with significant reduction in HMB from baseline. In addition, relugolix has been shown to have a possible reduction in pain and bulk symptoms compared with elagolix.[20]

Both GnRH agonists and antagonists are not reliable contraceptives and are contraindicated in pregnancy. Patients may use leuprolide with either hormonal or nonhormonal contraceptives (condom, spermicide). The use of hormonal contraception is not recommended with hormonal add-back combinations of elagolix or relugolix. Patients are advised to use nonhormonal contraceptives. Additionally, patients with contraindications to estrogen therapy are not candidates for GnRH antagonist add-back combination methods (Oriahnn or Myfembree).

### Progesterone Receptor Modulators

After the discovery that progesterone and progesterone receptors are essential for fibroid growth, selective progesterone receptor modulators (SPRMs) were studied for the treatment of fibroids.[21] The original SPRM, mifepristone, a progesterone antagonist, was initially commercialized for pregnancy termination and has recently been studied for treatment of fibroids. Ulipristal acetate (UPA), another SPRM commercialized for use as an emergency contraceptive, has also been studied for the treatment of fibroids. As a class, SPRMs have been shown to decrease menstrual blood loss and achieve amenorrhea. A Cochrane review of 14 randomized controlled trials (RCTs) concluded that short-term use of SPRMs results in improved quality of life, reduced menstrual bleeding, and higher rates of amenorrhea than placebo.[22] Despite their clear benefit on fibroid symptoms, the use of SPRMs has been limited by initial concerns owing to their unique effect on the endometrium, termed "progesterone receptor modulator–associated endometrial changes" or PAECs. These changes include thickening of the endometrium, cyst formation, and changes in gland cells and vascular cells. However, these changes have been found to be benign, not precancerous, and reversible.[21,23,24] Additionally, UPA has been associated with rare cases of serious liver toxicity, with some cases requiring liver transplantation.[11] Currently, UPA is only approved for use in Europe, for intermittent treatment of moderate to severe symptoms of fibroids before menopause and when surgical procedures (including UAE) are not possible or have failed. Underlying hepatic disorders are a contraindication to treatment, and liver function tests must be monitored before, during, and after treatment. An additional limitation to the use of mifepristone for treatment of fibroids is that a compounded formulation is required for doses suitable for treatment of this indication. Neither UPA nor mifepristone is presently FDA-approved for the treatment of fibroids.

## PROCEDURAL MANAGEMENT
### Uterine Artery Embolization

UAE is a minimally invasive, percutaneous, image-guided procedure that is performed by an interventional radiologist. The procedure is usually performed under intravenous conscious sedation and involves the catheterization and occlusion of the bilateral uterine arteries using particulate embolic agents, resulting in ischemic necrosis of the fibroids. Since its introduction in 1995, UAE has been associated with significant decrease in fibroid and uterine volume (by 50%–60%) that based on long-term follow-up data is maintained for up to 5 years.[25] Additionally, it is associated with improvement in HMB, bulk symptoms, and quality of life (80%–90%).[26] In fact, patient satisfaction and quality of life rating at 2 and 5 years after treatment are similar among patients undergoing UAE, myomectomy, or hysterectomy.[27] Advantages of UAE include that it is uterine sparing, short procedure and recovery time, decreased risk of transfusion when compared with myomectomy or hysterectomy, and is not limited by the number of fibroids or the patient's surgical history (intra-abdominal adhesions). Contraindications to UAE are pelvic inflammatory disease, gynecologic malignancy, and pregnancy. Relative contraindications include desire for future fertility, postmenopausal patients (due to risk of malignancy), severe renal insufficiency (contraindication to radiologic contrast agents), coagulopathy, and fibroid location (submucosal and pedunculated subserosal fibroids due to risk of intracavitary/intraperitoneal sloughing).[26]

The most common complication after UAE is postprocedure pain due to nonspecific ischemia of the uterus which often requires postoperative narcotics for pain management. Up to 40% of patients experience postembolization syndrome with diffuse abdominal pain, malaise, anorexia, nausea and vomiting, low-grade fever, and leukocytosis. This syndrome usually resolves within 48 hours, is self-limited, and usually only requires supportive therapy.[25] Overall complication rates after UAE as reported by the Society of Interventional Radiology are prolonged vaginal discharge 20%, transcervical expulsion of fibroids 15%, permanent amenorrhea 3% in patients younger than 45 years and 15% in those older than 45 years, 3% septicemia, and less than 1% for thromboembolism and nontarget embolization.[26] The most feared complication after UAE is intrauterine infection and, if untreated or refractory to antibiotics, can lead to sepsis and the need for hysterectomy. Despite significant initial success, rates of reintervention after UAE with hysterectomy, myomectomy, repeat embolization, medical management, or endometrial ablation are high. A Cochrane review found a five-fold increase in the likelihood of further intervention after UAE when compared with myomectomy or hysterectomy.[27] The EMMY trial, the largest randomized trial comparing UAE with hysterectomy, has published 10-year follow-up data demonstrating that 35% of patients who underwent a UAE ultimately required a hysterectomy. Despite this rate of intervention, 78% of subjects who underwent a UAE were very satisfied when compared with 87% who initially underwent a hysterectomy.[28]

The effect UAE may have on fertility and pregnancy is a topic of debate owing to the concern for potential adverse effects to ovarian reserve and endometrium. Compared with the general population, patients that have undergone a UAE seem to demonstrate higher rates of spontaneous abortion, preterm delivery, cesarean section, abnormal placentation, and postpartum hemorrhage. The degree to which confounding factors (advanced maternal age, prior infertility, and fibroid burden) contribute to these findings is unclear.[10,11]

In summary, UAE is a treatment option for patients with symptomatic fibroids who wish to avoid surgery or are poor surgical candidates. Patients that are considering further childbearing can undergo a UAE but require appropriate consultation regarding the pros and cons of the procedure and alternative therapies.

### High-Intensity Focused Ultrasound

HIFU is a uterine-sparing, percutaneous procedure that utilizes high-intensity ultrasound waves to ablate fibroids, thereby inducing coagulative necrosis. It is usually performed with conscious sedation as an outpatient procedure. Although this technique can be performed with either magnetic resonance–guided focused ultrasound (MRgFUS) or ultrasound guided focused ultrasound (USgFUS), only MRgFUS is currently FDA-approved.[10,29,30] MRI allows for real-time anatomic guidance and thermal monitoring for safe ablation.[31] Despite encouraging fertility and pregnancy reports, MRgFUS is best offered to premenopausal patients that do not desire future fertility. A recent systematic review of reproductive outcomes after MRgFUS reported a live birth rate of 73%. However, the outcomes data were heterogeneous and largely derived from retrospective analyses.[29]

Contraindications for HIFU treatment include pelvic inflammatory disease, gynecologic malignancy, and any contraindication to undergoing MRI (defibrillators, metal implants).[10] HIFU treatment works well with fibroids measuring 2 to 3 cm and has been successful with fibroids measuring less than 10 cm and uteri 20 to 24 weeks or smaller.[30] Additionally, factors such as tissue characteristics (T1 & T2 signal intensity, FIGO type) and technical limitations (scar tissue, abdominal subcutaneous fat, distance between fibroid and sacrum, bowel interposition between beam and fibroid) also dictate a patient's candidacy for this procedure.[32]

A recent single-center study of 252 patients undergoing MRgFUS reported significant symptom improvement in 74% of patients and a 12.7% reintervention rate.[31] Symptom relief and fibroid volume reduction rates are dependent on the volume of tissue that is not perfused (NPV) after treatment, and an NPV ratio of more than 80% has been suggested as a threshold for treatment success.[31] MRgFUS is a promising nonresective treatment approach for fibroids in patients that wish to avoid surgery; however, its effectiveness depends on careful patient selection.

## SURGICAL (NONRESECTIVE TREATMENT)
### Radiofrequency Fibroid Ablation

In recent years, radiofrequency ablation (RFA) of fibroids has been presented as a less invasive alternative to treating symptomatic fibroids. RFA was developed by adopting techniques used to treat solid tumors of the liver and adapting them to management of fibroids. RFA uses real-time ultrasound to identify the fibroids and apply radiofrequency energy from a handpiece using a laparoscopic or transcervical approach.[33] Ultrasound guidance allows placement of radiofrequency needles directly into the fibroid to target local treatment to only the fibroid tissue only. Radiofrequency fibroid ablation produces hyperthermic energy that induces coagulative necrosis of the fibroid. Once the fibroid undergoes coagulative necrosis, the process of fibroid resorption and volume reduction occurs over weeks to months depending on the fibroid size. A recent systematic review and meta-analysis of laparoscopic, vaginal, and transcervical RFA fibroid treatments by Bradley and colleagues reports health-related quality of life (HRQoL) scores increased by 39 points and Symptom Severity Score (SSS) decreased by 42 points. They also found a low annual cumulative reintervention rate of 4.2%, 8.2%, and 11.5% at 1, 2, and 3 years after ablation.[34] In addition to improved fibroid-related symptoms, RFA fibroid treatment also reduces fibroid volume. In a systematic review comparing RFA, UAE, and focused US treatments, RFA had the greatest reduction in mean fibroid volume compared with both UAE and MRgFUS. The pooled fibroid volume reductions at 6 month after treatment were as follows: RFA 70%, UAE 54%, FUS 32%.[35] Currently, there are two RFA modalities available for use in the U.S.: laparoscopic RFA (Lap-RFA) and transcervical RFA (TC-RFA).

Individuals who are considering RFA should be fully counseled about the risks of the procedure and the anticipated reduction in symptoms (further discussed in the later part of the article). It is important to have a good understanding of the anatomy of the uterus and associated fibroids before performing the procedure. In addition to standard of care preoperative evaluation for endometrial abnormalities with endometrial sampling, preoperative high-quality ultrasound or MRI is also recommended to map the location of the fibroids.

### Laparoscopic radiofrequency fibroid ablation

The first reported case of Lap-RFA was described by Lee in 2002.[33] The first device to be FDA-approved for the treatment of fibroids was the Acessa device (Hologic). The present system is called the Acessa ProVu system (**Fig. 2**). Lap-RFA requires an intra-abdominal ultrasound transducer (10 mm) that is placed directly on the uterine serosal surface to localize the fibroids. Next, the Acessa handpiece is introduced intra-abdominally and inserted directly into the fibroid where it delivers RF energy via a series of electrodes that can create ablation zones ranging from 1 cm to 6 cm (**Fig. 3**). The entire procedure is controlled with a single console and uses a tabletop field generator that produces a magnetic field detected by the guidance sensors in the handpiece. This system assists the surgeon in localizing the handpiece as it is introduced into the fibroid to maximize the ablation of the fibroid. Two return electrodes are placed on the legs of the patient. The FDA approval for the device is for patients with fibroids and a uterus less than 14-week size. Lap-RFA is capable of ablating fibroids in most anatomic positions, but is not recommended for FIGO types 0, 1, and

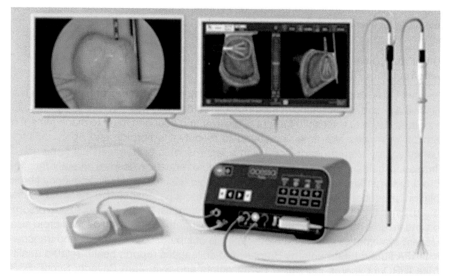

**Fig. 2.** Acessa ProVu system Equipment. (*Courtesy of* Hologic, Marlborough, MA; with permission.)

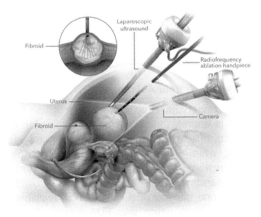

**Fig. 3.** Acessa ProVu system for laparoscopic RFA of fibroids demonstrated. (*Courtesy of Hologic, Marlborough, MA; with permission.*)

7. With clinical experience, larger fibroids and uteri can be treated in an off-label manner.

There have been several clinical trials that address the feasibility, safety, and ultimate long-term outcome of Lap-RFA. Thirty-one subjects involved in a single-site study with 1-year follow-up demonstrated that the procedure was safe and showed significant improvement in symptoms, with a 41% reduction in the mean uterine volume.[36] There was only one major complication from the procedure, an early postoperative vascular injury and hematoma of the abdominal wall that required a laparotomy that was believed to be a trocar injury, but an injury by the Lap-RFA needle could not be ruled out.

The Acessa device was ultimately approved by the FDA following a pivotal trial involving 135 subjects in a prospective trial with a 3-year follow-up period. The overall reintervention rate at 36 months was 11%.[37] The subjects were followed up using the Uterine Fibroid Symptom and Quality of Life (UFS-QOL) scoring system. There were statistically significant improvements in both symptom severity, decreasing from 60.2 at baseline to 27.6 at 3 years, and an increase in the quality of life score from 39.2 at baseline to 77.8 at 3 years. There are two RCTs that evaluate Lap-RFA with laparoscopic myomectomy.[38] In the first by Hahn and colleagues, fifty subjects were randomized 1:1 to laparoscopic myomectomy versus Lap-RFA with 12 months of follow-up. The study had intraoperative ultrasound to map the location of the fibroids before randomization as a strength. There was no statistical difference between the two procedures regarding improvement in the mean symptom scores and quality of life (UFS-QOL), demonstrating an overall equivalent outcome with Lap-RFA compared with the gold standard of therapy. However, subjects who underwent a myomectomy reported being very satisfied at a higher rate (86.5%) than (42.9%) those undergoing a Lap-RFA ($P = .004$), but in general, both therapies were well received. Additionally, two subjects who underwent a Lap-RFA subsequently conceived and subsequently delivered via healthy infants vaginal delivery.

The second trial was a randomized, postmarket, prospective multicenter, longitudinal study analyzing clinical outcomes and health care utilization.[39] The trial followed forty-five subjects, 23 in the Lap-RFA group and 22 in the laparoscopic myomectomy group for a period of 3 months. The Lap-RFA had a shorter hospital stay (6.7 hours vs 9.9 hours), had a shorter operative time (70 vs 86.5 minutes), and required fewer units of surgical equipment. At 3 months, the two treatments had similar reduction in symptoms scores and the combined per-patient direct and indirect costs were comparable. One myomectomy subject required overnight admission, and one Lap-RFA patient underwent a reintervention. The Lap-RFA subjects demonstrated a quicker return to work than the myomectomy subjects.

### Transcervical Radiofrequency Fibroid Ablation

TC-RFA offers a unique conservative fibroid treatment option because it allows for a vaginal procedure that is entirely "incision-free." Avoiding an incision on both the abdomen and the uterus offers the least invasive approach, faster recovery, and less intraperitoneal risk, while minimizing uterine risks such as the risk of uterine rupture, intrauterine adhesions (Asherman syndrome), abnormal placentation, and the potential need for cesarean delivery.[40] (**Fig. 4**)

Currently, there is only one transcervical RFA device available in the U.S., the Sonata® System (Gynesonics Inc.), which was FDA-approved in 2018 (**Fig. 5**). Unlike the Lap-RFA, which requires 3 incisions (1 for the laparoscope, 1 for the ultrasound probe, and 1 for the RF device), the TC-RFA procedure allows for an incisionless vaginal approach because the ultrasound probe and the RF device are both in the same hand-held TC-RFA instrument.[41,42] The device provides the operator with visual feedback as to the size of the ablation zone as well as the safety borders, which helps prevent unwanted thermal injury (**Fig. 6**). The TC-RFA device has a minimum and maximum ablation ring size (minimum: $2.0 \times 1.3$ cm and maximum: $5.0 \times 4.0$ cm). For fibroids larger than 5 cm, one may consider ablating multiple different areas within the same fibroid or decreasing the fibroid size preoperatively with Lupron before treatment.

TC-RFA has shown to be an effective minimally invasive treatment of symptomatic fibroids, reducing HMB in up to 95% of patients.[43] In this prospective, multicenter, single-arm transcervical ablation trial of 147 subjects, there was a very low 0.7% reintervention rate at 1 year, with 65% of patients reporting more than 50% reduction in bleeding and 62.4% fibroid volume reduction. Long-term improvements for fibroid-related symptoms have also been reported. Three-year follow-up results from the prospective SONATA Pivotal Trial also demonstrated a very high patient satisfaction rate (94%), decreased SSS (pre-RFA SSS $55 \pm 19$–$22 \pm 21$ at 3 years), increased HRQoL scores (pre-RFA HRQoL mean score 40 compared with 83 at 3 years), decreased work impairment from fibroids (51% pre-RFA to 12% at 3 years), and low reintervention rates (8.2%).[44] The longest longitudinal data available for TC-RFA were published in the VITALITY study, a retrospective study that reported an 11.8% surgical

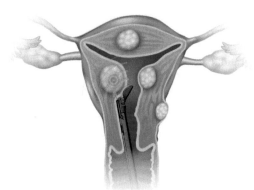

**Fig. 4.** Sonata system transcervical ablation demonstrated. (*Courtesy of* Gynesonics Inc., Redwood City, CA; with permission.)

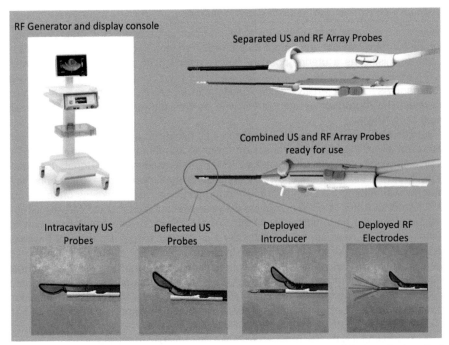

RF Generator and display console

Separated US and RF Array Probes

Combined US and RF Array Probes
ready for use

| Intracavitary US Probes | Deflected US Probes | Deployed Introducer | Deployed RF Electrodes |

**Fig. 5.** Sonata system detailed images of the components. (*Courtesy of* Gynesonics Inc., Redwood City, CA; with permission.)

reintervention rate over 64.4 months of follow up.[45] However, this study was limited by its small sample size (n = 17). Overall, TC-RFA seems to be an effective treatment with low reintervention rates of 0% to 4% at 1 year, 5% to 8% at 2 years, 8% to 11% at 3 years, and 11.8% at 5.4 years after treatment.[34,43–46] Additionally, the Fibroid Ablation Study-EU (FAST-EU) study reported a 67% fibroid volume reduction at 12 months.[41] These findings were maintained even among larger fibroids. In a subanalysis of the FAST-EU study, patients with fibroids larger than 5 cm demonstrated a 68% fibroid volume reduction 12 months after RFA treatment.[47] Additional studies support similar conclusions regarding reduction in fibroid volume after TC-RFA treatment.[43]

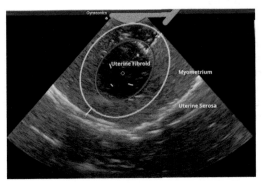

**Fig. 6.** Sonata system demonstration of ablation zone (*red*) and safety borders (*green*). (*Courtesy of* Gynesonics Inc., Redwood City, CA; with permission.)

### Pregnancy Outcomes and Radiofrequency Ablation

Review of the currently available literature on treatment efficacy and pregnancy outcomes for transcervical and laparoscopic radiofrequency ablation of uterine fibroids looks promising as a uterine-sparing, fertility-enabling treatment option. Currently, both Lap-RFA and TC-RFA are not approved by the US FDA as a fertility-enabling treatment. As a result, fertility-seeking patients have been excluded from RFA studies; however, the reproductive-age patient who desires future conception may benefit most from RFA.

Studies have analyzed post-RFA uterine wall thickness and intrauterine adhesion formation given the potential impact on pregnancy outcomes.[48,49] The INTEGRITY Trial, a large secondary analysis of the FAST-EU trial assessing the Sonata transcervical fibroid ablation system, showed there was no significant decrease in uterine wall integrity with little to no change in minimum myometrial wall thickness on follow-up MRI 12 months after TC-RFA compared with baseline measurements.[50] A prospective trial assessing the endometrial cavity after TC-RFA fibroid treatment with the Sonata system found no new intrauterine adhesions on hysteroscopic assessment 6 weeks after ablation compared with baseline hysteroscopy.[51] Six of these patients had opposing myomas, and none had new postablation adhesions. These studies suggest RFA fibroid treatment may potentially offer fertility benefits compared with standard myomectomy with favorable outcomes in terms of uterine wall thickness and adhesion formation. To our best knowledge, there have been no reported uterine ruptures following TC-RFA fibroid treatment.[52,53] However, given the rare incidence of uterine rupture, additional data are required to make any reliable conclusions.[51]

Subsequent pregnancies following TC-RFA trials show promising data for both safety and favorable reproductive outcomes.[53,54] A systematic review of all pregnancies reported after LSC-RFA and TC-RFA found 50 pregnancies among 923 RFA patients (40 among 559 LSC-RFAs and 10 among 364 TC-RFAs). Among the 50 who conceived, there were 6 spontaneous abortions (12%) and 44 full-term pregnancies (88%). Among the 44 deliveries, 24 were vaginal (54.5%) and 20 were cesarean (45.5%). There were no uterine ruptures, placenta accretas, or fetal complications, and the spontaneous abortion rate was comparable with the general obstetric population.[54]

RFA seems to be a safe option for reproductive-aged patients who desire future fertility and may offer potential fertility benefits compared with myomectomy in regards to uterine wall integrity and adhesion formation. Further research is needed to establish long-term outcomes for fibroid symptoms, fibroid volume reduction, and reproductive outcomes.

Lap-RFA and TC -RFA both represent new skills that require adequate training to become familiar with localization of the fibroids using an ultrasound being applied in a nonfamiliar manner. In addition, not all fibroids can be managed successfully with these technologies because both require careful attention to the zone of thermal injury produced by the devices to avoid injury to surrounding tissue. Introduction of these technologies should be done with appropriate training and observation until which time a clinician becomes comfortable with the localization process and the safe operation of the equipment.

### SUMMARY

Uterine fibroids are common and can significantly alter the quality of life of patients via abnormal bleeding, pressure sensation, and altered fertility. Previously, patients had a limited number of invasive procedures (myomectomy and hysterectomy) to treat their fibroids. The options for treatment have significantly increased in the last decade with the expanded use of UAE, HIFU, and the introduction of RFA and GnRH antagonists with combined add-back therapy. Clinicians who manage patients with fibroids now must become familiar with these new technologies to adequately counsel their patient or refer to someone who has expertise with fibroid management.

## CLINICS CARE POINTS

- Management and treatment of fibroids remains challenging because of the wide variety of sizes, locations, and symptoms associated with this pathology.
- Medical and nonresective treatment options represent advancements in the treatment of fibroids and should be offered to appropriate patients.
- Fibroid management should be carefully tailored to each individual patient to address fibroid symptoms while considering the patient's medical profile, family planning goals, age and risks.
- Managing fibroids among women who wish to conceive can be challenging because providers must balance optimal fibroid treatment with the patient's reproductive goals.

## DISCLOSURE

The authors have nothing to disclose.

## REFERENCES

1. Bulun SE. Uterine fibroids. N Engl J Med 2013;369(14):1344–55.
2. Munro MG, Critchley HOD, Broder MS, et al. FIGO classification system (PALM-COEIN) for causes of abnormal uterine bleeding in nongravid women of reproductive age. Int J Gynecol Obstet 2011;113(1):3–13.
3. Laughlin-Tommaso SK, Hesley GK, Hopkins MR, et al. Clinical limitations of the International Federation of Gynecology and Obstetrics (FIGO) classification of uterine fibroids. Int J Gynecol Obstet 2017;139(2):143–8.
4. Ghant MS, Sengoba KS, Recht H, et al. Beyond the physical: a qualitative assessment of the burden of symptomatic uterine fibroids on women's emotional and psychosocial health. J Psychosom Res 2015;78(5):499–503.
5. Cardozo ER, Clark AD, Banks NK, et al. The estimated annual cost of uterine leiomyomata in the United States. Am J Obstet Gynecol 2012;206(3):211.e1-9.
6. Giuliani E, As-Sanie S, Marsh EE. Epidemiology and management of uterine fibroids. Int J Gynaecol Obstet 2020;149(1):3–9.
7. Laughlin-Tommaso SK, Stewart EA. Moving Toward Individualized Medicine for Uterine Leiomyomas. Obstet Gynecol 2018;132(4):961–71.
8. Toro JR, Travis LB, Wu HJ, et al. Incidence patterns of soft tissue sarcomas, regardless of primary site, in the surveillance, epidemiology and end results program, 1978–2001: An analysis of 26,758 cases. Int J Cancer 2006;119(12):2922–30.
9. Uterine Morcellation for Presumed Leiomyomas: ACOG Committee Opinion, Number 822. Obstet Gynecol 2021;137(3):e63–74.
10. Laughlin-Tommaso SK. Non-surgical Management of Myomas. J Minim Invasive Gynecol 2018;25(2):229–36.
11. Management of Symptomatic Uterine Leiomyomas: ACOG Practice Bulletin, Number 228. Obstet Gynecol 2021;137(6):e100–15.

12. Bofill Rodriguez M, Lethaby A, Farquhar C. Non-steroidal anti-inflammatory drugs for heavy menstrual bleeding. Cochrane Database Syst Rev 2019;9(9): Cd000400.

13. Bryant-Smith AC, Lethaby A, Farquhar C, et al. Antifibrinolytics for heavy menstrual bleeding. Cochrane Database Syst Rev 2018;4(4):Cd000249.

14. Sinai Talaulikar V. Medical therapy for fibroids: An overview. Best Pract Res Clin Obstet Gynaecol 2018;46:48–56.

15. Lethaby A, Wise MR, Weterings MA, et al. Combined hormonal contraceptives for heavy menstrual bleeding. Cochrane Database Syst Rev 2019;2(2):Cd000154.

16. Curtis KM, Tepper NK, Jatlaoui TC, et al. U.S. medical eligibility criteria for contraceptive use, 2016. MMWR Recomm Rep 2016;65(3):1–103.

17. Matteson KA, Rahn DD, Wheeler TL 2nd, et al. Nonsurgical management of heavy menstrual bleeding: a systematic review. Obstet Gynecol 2013;121(3): 632–43.

18. Donnez J, Dolmans MM. Fibroids and medical therapy: bridging the gap from selective progesterone receptor modulators to gonadotropin-releasing hormone antagonist. Fertil Steril 2020;114(4):739–41.

19. Carr BR, Stewart EA, Archer DF, et al. Elagolix alone or with add-back therapy in women with heavy menstrual bleeding and uterine leiomyomas: a randomized controlled trial. Obstet Gynecol 2018;132(5):1252–64.

20. Al-Hendy A, Lukes AS, Poindexter AN 3rd, et al. Treatment of Uterine Fibroid Symptoms with Relugolix Combination Therapy. N Engl J Med 2021;384(7): 630–42.

21. Singh SS, Belland L, Leyland N, et al. The past, present, and future of selective progesterone receptor modulators in the management of uterine fibroids. Am J Obstet Gynecol 2018;218(6):563–72.e1.

22. Murji A, Whitaker L, Chow TL, et al. Selective progesterone receptor modulators (SPRMs) for uterine fibroids. Cochrane Database Syst Rev 2017;2017(4): CD010770.

23. Hartmann KE, Fonnesbeck C, Surawicz T, et al. AHRQ Comparative Effectiveness Reviews. In: Management of uterine fibroids. Rockville (MD): Agency for Healthcare Research and Quality (US); 2017.

24. Donnez J, Dolmans MM. Uterine fibroid management: from the present to the future. Hum Reprod Update 2016;22(6):665–86.

25. SOGC clinical practice guidelines. Uterine fibroid embolization (UFE). Number 150, October 2004. Int J Gynaecol Obstet 2005;89(3):305–18.

26. Silberzweig JE, Powell DK, Matsumoto AH, et al. Management of Uterine Fibroids: A Focus on Uterine-sparing Interventional Techniques. Radiology 2016; 280(3):675–92.

27. Gupta JK, Sinha A, Lumsden MA, et al. Uterine artery embolization for symptomatic uterine fibroids. Cochrane Database Syst Rev 2014;12:Cd005073.

28. De Bruijn AM, Ankum WM, Reekers JA, et al. Uterine artery embolization vs hysterectomy in the treatment of symptomatic uterine fibroids: 10-year outcomes from the randomized EMMY trial. Am J Obstet Gynecol 2016;215(6):745.e1-2.

29. Anneveldt KJ, Van 'T Oever HJ, Nijholt IM, et al. Systematic review of reproductive outcomes after High Intensity Focused Ultrasound treatment of uterine fibroids. Eur J Radiol 2021;141:109801.

30. Hesley GK, Gorny KR, Woodrum DA. MR-Guided Focused Ultrasound for the Treatment of Uterine Fibroids. CardioVascular Interv Radiol 2013;36(1):5–13.

31. Mindjuk I, Trumm CG, Herzog P, et al. MRI predictors of clinical success in MR-guided focused ultrasound (MRgFUS) treatments of uterine fibroids: results from a single centre. Eur Radiol 2015;25(5):1317–28.

32. Duc NM, Keserci B. Review of influential clinical factors in reducing the risk of unsuccessful MRI-guided HIFU treatment outcome of uterine fibroids. Diagn Interv Radiol 2018;24(5):283–91.

33. Lee BB, Yu SP. Radiofrequency Ablation of Uterine Fibroids: a Review. Curr Obstet Gynecol Rep 2016;5(4):318–24.

34. Bradley LD, Pasic RP, Miller LE. Clinical Performance of Radiofrequency Ablation for Treatment of Uterine Fibroids: Systematic Review and Meta-Analysis of Prospective Studies. J Laparoendoscopic Adv Surg Tech 2019;29(12):1507–17.

35. Taheri M, Galo L, Potts C, et al. Nonresective treatments for uterine fibroids: a systematic review of uterine and fibroid volume reductions. Int J Hyperthermia 2019; 36(1):295–301.

36. Garza Leal JG, Hernandez Leon I, Castillo Saenz L, et al. Laparoscopic ultrasound-guided radiofrequency volumetric thermal ablation of symptomatic uterine leiomyomas: feasibility study using the Halt 2000 Ablation System. J Minim Invasive Gynecol 2011;18(3):364–71.

37. Berman JM, Guido RS, Garza Leal JG, et al. Three-year outcome of the Halt trial: a prospective analysis of radiofrequency volumetric thermal ablation of myomas. J Minim Invasive Gynecol 2014;21(5):767–74.

38. Hahn M, Brucker S, Kraemer D, et al. Radiofrequency Volumetric Thermal Ablation of Fibroids and Laparoscopic Myomectomy: Long-Term Follow-up From a Randomized Trial. Geburtshilfe und Frauenheilkunde 2015;75(05):442–9.

39. Rattray DD, Weins L, Regush LC, et al. Clinical outcomes and health care utilization pre- and post-laparoscopic radiofrequency ablation of symptomatic fibroids and laparoscopic myomectomy: a randomized trial of uterine-sparing techniques (TRUST) in Canada. Clinicoecon Outcomes Res 2018;10:201–12.

40. Aarts JW, Nieboer TE, Johnson N, et al. Surgical approach to hysterectomy for benign gynaecological disease. Cochrane Database Syst Rev 2015;8: CD003677.

41. Brölmann H, Bongers M, Garza-Leal JG, et al. The FAST-EU trial: 12-month clinical outcomes of women after intrauterine sonography-guided transcervical radiofrequency ablation of uterine fibroids. Gynecol Surg 2016;13:27–35.

42. Brooks EA, Singer AM, Delvadia DR, et al. The CHOICES Study: Facility Level Comparative Cost, Resource Utilization, and Outcomes Analysis of Myomectomy Compared to Transcervical Fibroid Ablation. Clinicoecon Outcomes Res 2020;12: 299–306.

43. Chudnoff S, Guido R, Roy K, et al. Ultrasound-Guided Transcervical Ablation of Uterine Leiomyomas. Obstet Gynecol 2019;133(1):13–22.

44. Lukes A, Green MA. Three-Year Results of the SONATA Pivotal Trial of Transcervical Fibroid Ablation for Symptomatic Uterine Myomata. J Gynecol Surg 2020; 36(5):228–33.

45. Garza-Leal JG. Long-Term Clinical Outcomes of Transcervical Radiofrequency Ablation of Uterine Fibroids: The VITALITY Study. J Gynecol Surg 2019;35(1): 19–23.

46. Miller CE, Osman KM. Transcervical Radiofrequency Ablation of Symptomatic Uterine Fibroids: 2-Year Results of the SONATA Pivotal Trial. J Gynecol Surg 2019;35(6):345–9.

47. Shifrin G, Engelhardt M, Gee P, et al. Transcervical fibroid ablation with the Sonata™ system for treatment of submucous and large uterine fibroids. Int J Gynaecol Obstet 2021;155(1):79–85.
48. Parker WH, Einarsson J, Istre O, et al. Risk factors for uterine rupture after laparoscopic myomectomy. J Minim Invasive Gynecol 2010;17(5):551–4.
49. Sizzi O, Rossetti A, Malzoni M, et al. Italian multicenter study on complications of laparoscopic myomectomy. J Minim Invasive Gynecol 2007;14(4):453–62.
50. Bongers M, Gupta J, Garza-Leal JG, et al. The INTEGRITY Trial: Preservation of Uterine-Wall Integrity 12 Months After Transcervical Fibroid Ablation with the Sonata System. J Gynecol Surg 2019;35(5):299–303.
51. Bongers M, Quinn SD, Mueller MD, et al. Evaluation of uterine patency following transcervical uterine fibroid ablation with the Sonata system (the OPEN clinical trial). Eur J Obstet Gynecol Reprod Biol 2019;242:122–5.
52. Keltz J, Levie M, Chudnoff S. Pregnancy Outcomes After Direct Uterine Myoma Thermal Ablation: Review of the Literature. J Minim Invasive Gynecol 2017; 24(4):538–45.
53. Khaw SC, Anderson RA, Lui MW. Systematic review of pregnancy outcomes after fertility-preserving treatment of uterine fibroids. Reprod Biomed Online 2020; 40(3):429–44.
54. Polin M, Hur H-C. Radiofrequency ablation of uterine fibroids and pregnancy outcomes: an updated review of the literature. J Minimally Invasive Gynecol 2022.

# Office Hysteroscopy
## Setting up Your Practice for Success

Anna Zelivianskaia, MD[a],*, James K. Robinson III, MD, MS[b]

## KEYWORDS

- Office • Outpatient • Intrauterine adhesions • Asherman syndrome • Hysteroscopy
- Abnormal uterine bleeding

## KEY POINTS

- Hysteroscopy is the gold standard for the evaluation of abnormal uterine bleeding and intrauterine pathology. With advances in hysteroscope size and operative instruments, office hysteroscopy has become more practical and effective.
- Vaginoscopy is a hysteroscopic technique without a speculum or tenaculum with the greatest patient comfort and lowest pain levels.
- Many types of instruments and sterilization methods are available for the office hysteroscopy practice with unique cost-benefit factors.
- General anesthesia is not required, and minimal medication can be used for adequate pain control in office hysteroscopy, particularly with the vaginoscopy technique.
- The decreased costs of office hysteroscopy compared with the operating room setting have been demonstrated, but reimbursement challenges still exist.

 Video content accompanies this article at http://www.obgyn.theclinics.com.

## INTRODUCTION

Hysteroscopy is a minimally invasive method of assessing the uterine cavity and addressing pathology. The procedure was first performed in 1869 and office hysteroscopy began in the 1980s.[1] Advancements in technology allowing for smaller instruments and lower costs have allowed office hysteroscopy to become more practical.[1,2]

Hysteroscopy is the gold standard for the diagnosis of abnormal uterine bleeding.[3] Hysteroscopy with tissue sampling has lower false positives and false negative rates than endometrial biopsy, blind dilation and curettage, hysterosalpingography, or

---

[a] Department of Obstetrics and Gynecology, MedStar Washington Hospital Center, Georgetown University School of Medicine, 110 Irving Street, Washington, DC 20010, USA; [b] Women's and Infants' Services, Minimally Invasive Gynecologic Surgery, MedStar Washington Hospital Center, 106 Irving Street, Northwest Suite 405 South, Washington, DC 20010, USA
* Corresponding author.
*E-mail addresses:* Anna.S.Zelivianskaia@medstar.net (A.Z.); James.K.Robinson@medstar.net (J.K.R.)

Obstet Gynecol Clin N Am 49 (2022) 315–327
https://doi.org/10.1016/j.ogc.2022.02.011
0889-8545/22/© 2022 Elsevier Inc. All rights reserved.

obgyn.theclinics.com

ultrasound techniques.[3] Ultrasound is limited in delineating endometrial thickening from other intrauterine lesions.[4] While saline infusion sonogram (SIS) can better distinguish endometrial thickening from other pathology compared with routine ultrasound, SIS is also painful and has limitations in the identification of pathology specifics.[4] For example, SIS cannot distinguish a cluster of polyps from a submucosal leiomyoma. Hysteroscopy provides a more comprehensive evaluation and misses less than 0.5% of serious pathology.[3] One study noted the sensitivity of ultrasound, SIS, and office hysteroscopy to be 56%, 81%, and 87%, respectively.[5] The specificity of these three modalities was 72%, 100%, and 100%, respectively.[5] Hysteroscopy is also superior for the identification of focal lesions causing abnormal uterine bleeding when compared with either ultrasound or endometrial biopsy.[6] Removal of endometrial polyps under direct visualization is preferable to blind curettage, which is lower in accuracy and may not remove the entire lesion.[7]

### Indications and Efficacy

Indications for hysteroscopy are described in **Box 1**. There is substantial overlap in the indications for office or outpatient surgery hysteroscopy. This list is not exhaustive and other reasons may exist in individualized patient scenarios. Posttreatment follow-up is a broad indication that can apply to follow-up for various medical or surgical treatments. For example, hysteroscopy can be performed after tamoxifen use to evaluate for malignancy or after a myomectomy or septoplasty to evaluate for intrauterine adhesions.[6] Indications for removal of polyps or fibroids via operative hysteroscopy are abnormal uterine bleeding, infertility, or recurrent pregnancy loss.[7] Indications for intrauterine adhesiolysis are secondary amenorrhea, irregular menstruation, or imaging evidence of adhesions in women pursuing fertility.[7]

Hysteroscopy is a safe and effective tool for the identification and treatment of the intrauterine pathology described above. The success of hysteroscopic myomectomy, usually performed in the operating room, is dependent on the type of fibroid, but

---

**Box 1**
**Indications for hysteroscopy**

- Abnormal uterine bleeding
- Cesarean scar defect (Isthmocele)
- Foreign body or intracavitary mass
  - Endometrial polyp
  - Submucosal fibroid(s)
  - Retained products of conception
  - Cystic adenomyosis
  - Imbedded IUD or IUD with a lost string
- Endometrial thickening
- Infertility
- Implantation difficulties or recurrent pregnancy loss
- Suspected or known congenital vaginal, cervical, and/or uterine Mullerian anomaly
- Suspected or known intrauterine adhesions
- Posttreatment follow-up
- Preoperative planning
- Vaginal lesions in patients that cannot tolerate a speculum examination

overall success rates are quite high for fibroids of which greater than 50% are within the cavity. Staged resections may be required for large submucosal fibroids.[7] Success rates of hysteroscopic lysis of adhesions, performed in either the operating room or office setting, are also high and ranges from 88% to 95%.[8,9] Reformation of adhesions is possible but does not occur in most women. Prevention strategies for recurrent adhesions are outside the scope of this article.

## See and Treat Approach in Office Hysteroscopy

Diagnostic hysteroscopy includes a visual assessment of the uterine cavity to note any visual pathology. Operative hysteroscopy allows for the ability to treat any observed pathology. There is significant overlap in indications for diagnostic and operative procedures and if a procedure is started with diagnostic intent, the "see and treat" approach can be used.[4] The "see and treat" approach allows a seamless transition from diagnostic to operative hysteroscopy if abnormal pathology is noted and the patient continues to tolerate the procedure.[4] Assuming proper set-up and instrumentation availability, this technique allows for the fewest number of interventions for proper patient care. Both diagnostic and operative office hysteroscopy procedures have high success rates with a meta-analysis showing the overall success of diagnostic hysteroscopy to be 96.6%.[10] A large retrospective review found successful completion of diagnostic office hysteroscopy in more than 97% of attempted cases.[11] The same study demonstrated that immediate treatment by polypectomy was possible in more than 65% of cases whereby diagnostic hysteroscopy was successful, and an endometrial polyp was identified.[11] Factors associated with successful concomitant treatment were younger age, lower BMI, and smaller polyp size.[11] A randomized control trial comparing office polypectomy to removal in the OR found one woman out of 20 randomized to the office arm was not able to complete the procedure due to cervical stenosis.[12,13] All other procedures were successful and office hysteroscopy had decreased pain and increased satisfaction.[12]

## Discussion of Hysteroscopy in the Office Practice Setting

### Patient selection and preparation

There are few contraindications to office hysteroscopy, which include pregnancy, active pelvic inflammatory disease, or active herpetic or human papilloma virus infections, and are the same contraindications to performing hysteroscopy in the operating room. However, selecting the appropriate patient for the procedure is important.[6] Similar to hysteroscopy in the operating room, informed consent must be obtained before the procedure. Information on the size and location of intracavitary pathology, anticipated resection time, and physician expertise should all be considered. Additional criteria for patient selection in the office are partly dependent on the need for conscious sedation or another type of anesthesia. For example, patients with comorbidities such as sleep apnea may not be good candidates for office hysteroscopy requiring conscious sedation without an anesthesia team present.[7] Additionally, patients with significant anxiety or a history of a failed office procedure may not be good candidates for this setting. In randomized trials with appropriately selected patients, office hysteroscopy was preferred when compared with the operating room.[7] Office hysteroscopy was associated with higher patient satisfaction and faster recovery time.[7]

No significant workup is required before an office hysteroscopy procedure, but a pregnancy test immediately before the procedure is necessary.[7] Office hysteroscopy should ideally be performed during the early proliferative phase of the cycle, shortly after menstruation, to achieve the best visualization of the cavity.[8] In patients where menstrual timing is challenging, performing the procedure after a progestin withdrawal or after 3 weeks of continuous progestational therapy is also effective. No antibiotic prophylaxis is indicated before hysteroscopy procedures.[8]

### Instruments

The 5 key components of an office hysteroscopy set-up are the hysteroscope, endo-camera, monitor, light source, and light cable.[14] Most of the hysteroscopes currently in use for diagnostic and/or operative procedures have continuous flow with an operating channel that allow for the insertion of instruments.[14] The development of hysteroscopes with smaller diameters have made these procedures more comfortable and more likely to be performed with little or no anesthesia, as discussed later in discussion.

Hysteroscopes can be either reusable or disposable (**Table 1**). Within these categories, hysteroscopes can be further divided into the following: flexible, hystero-fiberscopes, and rigid rod lens. Hystero-fiberscopes are rarely used because they are costly, not durable, and difficult to sterilize.[14] We will limit our discussion to flexible and rigid hysteroscopes.

Reusable or disposable semirigid instruments that are commonly used for operative office hysteroscopy include scissors, grasping or biopsy forceps, tenacula, and polyp snares. Scissors are useful for lysing intrauterine adhesions and undermining various pathologies, such as polyps, small submucosal fibroids, or retained products of conception. Biopsy forceps are intended for tissue sampling. Pathology extraction is often facilitated by the utilization of grasping forceps, tenaculum, or snare.

5 French (Fr) monopolar and bipolar wire tip electrodes can also be used in the office but require the use of a radiofrequency generator, appropriate distention media, and a formal fluid management system to accurately follow fluid deficit. More recently, a 5 mm bipolar office-resectoscope was developed which allows the use of 15 Fr loop, wire, and coagulation tips (Karl Storz) for true resectoscopic surgery often without cervical dilation. Similarly, multiple small gauge tissue morcellators are also on the market that can be used without cervical dilation in selected patients (see **Table 1**).

### Distention media

There are several types of distention media used for hysteroscopy, including high viscosity fluid, low viscosity fluid, and gas. High viscosity media has the advantage of not mixing with blood, which facilitates the evaluation of the uterine cavity in the presence of bleeding.[15] The most commonly used high-viscosity fluid for uterine distention is a hyperosmolar solution of 32% dextran 70 in 10% glucose.[15] However, the high osmolality of this fluid can lead to cardiovascular issues and pulmonary edema at relatively low volumes.[15] Due to the risk of adverse events and the tendency of dextran 70 to caramelize on instruments if not immediately cleaned, it is not a media commonly used for hysteroscopy.[15]

The most used media for distention in office hysteroscopy is saline, a low viscosity electrolyte-rich solution. This is a relatively safe solution that is used with bipolar energy and does not cause electrolyte imbalance but can cause fluid overload and pulmonary edema if absorbed in very large quantities.[15] This risk is extremely low with short office procedures. Lactated ringer's is presumed to have the same qualities but has not been specifically tested in the office hysteroscopy setting.[15] Electrolyte-poor solution, such as 1.5% glycine, 5% mannitol, or 3% sorbitol, is required if monopolar energy is used. The use of monopolar energy is less common in office hysteroscopy than bipolar energy. These electrolyte-poor solutions are also low viscosity

**Table 1**
Disposable office hysteroscopy equipment

| Product | Disposable | Diagnostic | Operative | OD (mm) | Instruments | One Time Cost | Per Use Cost | Notes |
|---|---|---|---|---|---|---|---|---|
| Myosure Manual | Partial | X | X | 3.7–6 | Manual Tissue Removal Device | Scope $9655 | Device $550 | Tissue Removal Device is disposable |
| Benesta Hysteroscope | Partial | X | X | 5.8 | Disposable tissue Removal Device with 15 mm cutting window | Scope $3753 | | |
| Lina OperaScope | Yes | x | x | 4.2 | Biopsy forceps, Rat tooth, scissors, Lasso (10 and 16 mm), Angled Lasso (10 and 16 mm) | N/A | $258 | Operative instruments range $49–149 |
| EndoSee Advance | Partial | x | x | 4.3 | Biopsy forceps, scissors, Alligator grasper, Spoon | $2995 for reusable Scope bundle | $175 | Single use semi flexible cannula. Reusable handpiece and monitor |
| Luminelle 360 | Partial | x | x | 3.7–5.7 | Dilating rotosheath | $3000 for reusable Scope; $4500 for reusable Scope bundle | $99–150 | Reusable scope, Single use dilating rotosheath |
| Aveta System | Yes | x | x | 4.6 | Aveta Auto Morcellator | N/A | Opal scope $150 Coral Scope $250 Auto resector $450 | Suction within the handle, tissue container attached, auto morcellation with 7 mm cutting window |

and provide excellent visualization but can affect the systemic sodium balance if absorbed in large quantities.[15] Excessive fluid absorption will lead to hyponatremia, which can cause cerebral edema and other neurologic issues.[15]

Carbon dioxide ($CO_2$) is another option used historically because it is generally well-tolerated and does not distort the view of the uterine cavity.[14] However, $CO_2$ can lead to uterine spasm, subdiaphragmatic irritation, or embolism in rare cases. Recent literature suggests that electrolyte-rich fluid is the preferred distention media, especially during operative procedures, as the continuous inflow and outflow can clear blood, clots, and debris.[3,14] Saline has lower costs compared with $CO_2$ and allows for the use of bipolar instruments.

Distention media can be delivered using atmospheric pressure, a "squeeze bag" pressure system, or an electronically controlled fluid management system.[14] We use a pressure bag set-up (**Fig. 1**). This type of setup is more economical than a complete fluid management system but does not allow the exact measurement of how much fluid the patient has absorbed. Fluid can leave the uterus by the outflow channel, leakage from the cervix or fallopian tubes, or extravasation.[16] The primary mechanism of systemic fluid absorption during hysteroscopy is through extravasation via venous sinuses in the endometrium and myometrium.[15] While the inability to precisely measure fluid inflow and outflow is a limitation, absorption of clinically relevant volumes of fluid distention media is a rare occurrence in office hysteroscopy whereby mechanical or radiofrequency resectoscopic procedures are not being used. Additionally, one can conservatively limit fluid intake by using a 1L fluid bag for the procedure. When more advanced resectoscopic techniques are used, a formal fluid management system is a necessity.

### Sterilization or high-level disinfection

Sterilization refers to the destruction of all microbial life, while high-level disinfection uses an enzymatic agent to destroy all recognized pathogenic microbes but not necessarily all types of microorganisms such as bacterial endospores that might be present on inanimate objects.

Gas sterilization using either ethylene oxide gas or vaporized hydrogen peroxide gas plasma (STERRAD) are the techniques most compatible with reusable rigid and flexible hysteroscopes. Gas sterilization can be performed at a well-equipped clinic location or at an off-site facility using a medical equipment transport service. High-level

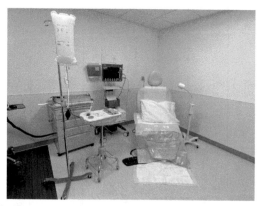

**Fig. 1.** Example of office hysteroscopy room setup. A pressure bag system and drape to catch fluid are used.

disinfection, using an enzymatic solution, can be performed in most office settings without a significant financial investment. Several considerations should be considered before committing to a preferred processing solution.

Before processing reusable instruments, the hysteroscope must be taken apart and any soiled areas wiped down. Then the hysteroscope should be cleaned with hot water and the lumen flushed with distilled water. Lenses should be buffed immediately after use. Alternatively, water and a detergent cleaning solution can be used in this precleaning step.[17] The hysteroscope can then be processed using the approved technique according to manufacturer instructions. This is usually accomplished with either autoclave, the highest level of sterilization, or high-level disinfecting enzymatic solution. The latter is more cost-effective but may not comply with specific institutional requirements.

If using an enzymatic solution, it should be diluted according to label instructions and the hysteroscope soaked for 5 to 15 minutes.[17–19] Several kinds of enzymatic solutions are on the market, including Steris Prolystica and Cidex OPA solutions.[19,20] The device and components should then be scrubbed and rinsed under hot water, followed by a rinse with purified water.[18] If gas sterilization is used, the scrub and rinse steps should be completed first.[18] Alternatively, rigid hysteroscopes and instruments can be sterilized in the autoclave at 134°C.[17] After sterilization or high-level disinfection is complete, the instruments must be packaged carefully to maintain sterility.[17]

### Vaginoscopy versus traditional hysteroscopy technique

For any type of hysteroscopy, the patient should be positioned in the dorsal lithotomy position, taking care to avoid unnecessary pressure that may cause nerve injury. It is helpful to perform a bimanual examination before the procedure to assess the position of the uterus. Patients are usually most comfortable if asked to void before the procedure. The hysteroscope needs to be set up, the camera white-balanced and focused, and the inflow tract primed (see **Fig. 1**; **Figs. 2–4**).

With the traditional technique, a speculum is first inserted. The cervix is visualized and grasped anteriorly with a single-tooth tenaculum or allis clamp.[1] The cervix is then dilated, if necessary, to the diameter of the hysteroscope being used and the hysteroscope is then inserted.[1] At the same time, counter traction is applied with the tenaculum to straighten the uterus.[1]

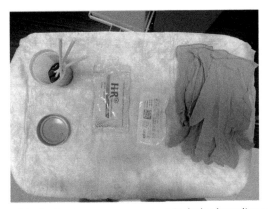

**Fig. 2.** Preparatory table for hysteroscopy procedure includes betadine solution, lubricant, and gloves.

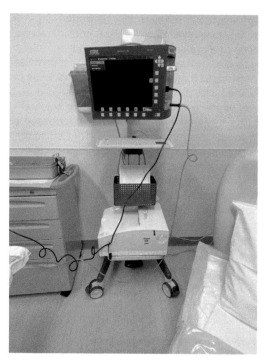

**Fig. 3.** Video monitor, light source, and printer.

With the vaginoscopic entry or no-touch technique, the need for the traditional instruments used for entry, such as a speculum or cervical tenaculum, is avoided. The provider begins vaginoscopy by introducing the hysteroscope with distention fluid flowing into the vagina (**Fig. 4**). The posterior fornix is easily identified, and the scope is advanced upwards to identify the external os. Once the cervix is located, the hysteroscope is carefully inserted and passed through the internal os into the uterine cavity under direct visualization. Distention media is flowing throughout these steps to expand the cervical canal and cavity.[1–7] If entry is challenging, the uterus can be brought to a more axial position by applying pressure above the pubic symphysis or

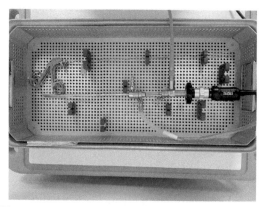

**Fig. 4.** Sterile rigid hysteroscope and reusable instruments.

anterior pressure digitally through the rectum.[7] Full bladder distention will also reduce uterine anteflexion. Multiple studies have shown there is no difference in failed procedures when comparing vaginoscopy to the traditional hysteroscopic technique.[7] Vaginoscopy leads to significantly decreased pain, as described further in the next section.[16] (Video 1).

In patients with a nulliparous or stenotic cervix, placement of a speculum for the dilation of the external cervical os followed by removal of the speculum before the placement of the hysteroscope is often sufficient to allow the utilization of the better tolerated vaginoscopic technique.

### Pain management

The office hysteroscopy experience begins with entry into the examination room and mitigation of patient anxiety is a vital component. Efficient room setup and calming techniques, such as music or dim lighting, can alleviate patient anxiety and reduce the perception of pain.[21] Constant communication during the procedure leads to a more positive perception of the procedure during office hysteroscopy and may lower anxiety levels.[22]

There are multiple studies describing office hysteroscopy performed without analgesia, even with the use of bipolar electrocautery.[11,23] Sensory innervation is largely absent in endometrium, polyps, adhesions, and myomas. In one large study, the mean pain score during office hysteroscopy was 3.57 out of 10.[6] The mean pain levels with no-touch vaginoscopy are significantly lower compared with the traditional technique utilizing a speculum and cervical stabilizing instruments.[25] Smaller hysteroscopes, less than 5 mm, are also associated with decreased pain. One randomized control trial showed lower pain levels with a 3.5 mm hysteroscope compared with either a 5 mm hysteroscope or a 5 mm hysteroscope with paracervical block.[24] Factors associated with higher levels of perceived pain include cervical stenosis, postmenopausal status, anxiety, and chronic pelvic pain.[24]

Premedication with nonsteroidal anti-inflammatory drugs (NSAIDs) or opioids, such as tramadol or oxycodone, can also reduce discomfort. Administration of 800 mg ibuprofen 2 hours before the procedure has been shown to decrease patient discomfort.[1] A meta-analysis of studies comparing NSAID use to control groups showed a statistically significant decrease in reported pain levels during and after office hysteroscopy.[25] Opioid use 40 to 60 minutes before the procedure was also associated with decreased pain scores during and after office hysteroscopy compared with control groups.[25] Two studies reported a decrease in procedural pain with oral antispasmodic use 1 hour before the procedure compared with a control.[25] However, there was a statistically significant increase in adverse events with use of either opioids or antispasmodics.[25] One large study compared transcutaneous electrical nerve stimulation (TENS) against a control group for office hysteroscopy and showed a statistically significant pain reduction and no increase in adverse events.[25] Virtual reality headsets with a calming meditation application were subjectively well received by patients but did not show a significant decrease in objectively rated pain during office hysteroscopy with a vaginoscopic approach.[26]

Warming the saline distention media or adding ropivacaine or levobupivacaine can lower discomfort during the procedure. Paracervical block has been shown to decrease pain with tenaculum placement and cervical dilation,[7,11] but if vaginoscopy is used without the need for cervical dilation paracervical block is not helpful for pain management and increases the risk of a vasovagal reaction.

There is currently insufficient evidence to recommend routine cervical ripening. The use of vaginal misoprostol before the procedure can reduce pain during access in select women.[7] Misoprostol is a prostaglandin E1 analog and various dosages of misoprostol have been studied. A dose of 200 to 400mcg intravaginally is the most common dose if cervical ripening is desired.[7] Its use must be balanced with adverse effects of the medication, including abdominal cramping, increased body temperature, and vaginal bleeding.[7] One meta-analysis examining the effects of misoprostol showed that cervical dilation, cervical lacerations, and creation of false passage were significantly reduced after vaginal misoprostol administration.[27] These positive effects were not seen with oral or sublingual misoprostol administration.[27] In a subgroup analysis of diagnostic hysteroscopy, there was a lower need for cervical dilation, but it was not statistically significant.[27] If a need for cervical dilation is expected, it may be reasonable to pretreat with vaginal misoprostol to improve patient comfort and lower complications.

### Economic challenges

Successful office hysteroscopy procedures have lower costs compared with similar procedures performed in the operating room due to lower anesthesia and facility costs. Additionally, from the patient perspective, women appreciate decreased procedure costs, faster recovery, and less time off work with less associated lost income.[6,24] However, several economic challenges to wider adoption of office hysteroscopy exist, including total costs and reimbursement in the office setting.

There is convincing evidence that if hysteroscopy can be accomplished in the office it is more cost-effective than performing the same procedure in the operating room. One study compared average costs of office hysteroscopy procedure with local anesthetic to OR hysteroscopy with either general anesthesia or local anesthetic and found considerable cost savings.[28] The cost for the office procedure was $482 compared with $716 and $1482 for OR hysteroscopy with local anesthetic and general anesthesia, respectively.[28] Decreased staff costs were the primary factor for cost savings.[28] A meta-analysis of office hysteroscopy compared with OR hysteroscopy also showed significantly decreased costs for the office procedures.[29] Specifically, the OR hysteroscopy cost range was $268 to 3144 and the office procedure cost range was $97 to 1258.[29]

In the last several years, the cost-effectiveness of office procedures has been recognized and reimbursement has increased, but this has not been universal for all types of office hysteroscopy. The relative value units (RVUs) associated with physician services are determined by the Medicare Resource-Based Relative Value Scale. Based on this system, certain office procedures are valued at a much higher relative value than others. For example, since 2017, a hysteroscopic polypectomy earns 6.71 RVUs in a facility but 38.51 RVUs if performed in the office.[9] This translates to an additional monetary reimbursement of approximately $1100.[9] It is important to know whether an office practice charges a facility fee as this may decrease reimbursement even if the procedure is not performed in the OR. Other types of hysteroscopies do not have a set amount of RVUs for the office setting and thus do not have the same significant monetary difference in reimbursement. For hysteroscopic lysis of intrauterine adhesions and hysteroscopic myomectomies, there is less than a $10 difference for a procedure performed in the office compared with a facility.[9] There is a moderate difference in reimbursement for diagnostic hysteroscopy in the office, which earns an additional 3.2 RVUs translating to an additional $115 in reimbursement amount per procedure.[9]

The decision to invest in reusable equipment as compared with disposable equipment must take many factors into consideration. Disposable instruments are convenient and do not require a significant capital investment or sterilization.

Unfortunately, the cost of the disposables also cuts into reimbursement fees significantly. A busy office hysteroscopy practice can typically recoup capital investments for reusable instruments after approximately 50 office procedures.[10] Service agreements can also be purchased with all the major equipment suppliers as insurance against breakage, repair, and replacement which can be valuable. In general, it makes economic sense to use disposable equipment in a low-volume setting and reusable equipment in a high-volume setting. Given the wide range of indications for office hysteroscopy, most busy gynecology practices will be able to build a high-volume program without much difficulty. **Table 1** highlights some important cost considerations.

## SUMMARY

Office hysteroscopy is a safe and effective method for the diagnosis and treatment of a wide range of intrauterine pathology. Unfortunately, it is underutilized, and this review aims to describe the building blocks of a successful practice. Office hysteroscopy is well-tolerated with minimal premedication, but proper patient selection and preparation are important. Additionally, using the vaginoscopy technique is better tolerated by patients with similar success rates. Recent improvements in procedural work RVUs incentivize the adoption of the technology. While economic and sterilization challenges exist, there are numerous options available that make the incorporation of office hysteroscopy in most busy gynecology practices both viable and profitable.

## CLINICS CARE POINTS

- Office hysteroscopy is a safe and effective method for the diagnosis and treatment of various intrauterine pathologies, including abnormal uterine bleeding and infertility.
- Proper patient selection and preparation is crucial, but preprocedure workup is minimal and requires a pregnancy test.
- Many types of hysteroscope types exist and can be classified as either reusable or disposable.
- Office hysteroscopy can be accomplished with little to no anesthesia and the vaginoscopy technique leads to lower pain levels compared with traditional hysteroscopy.
- A successful and cost-effective office practice can be built with a thorough knowledge of reimbursement structures, equipment types, and sterilization methods available.

## DISCLOSURE

The authors have nothing to disclose.

## SUPPLEMENTARY DATA

Supplementary data related to this article can be found online at https://doi.org/10.1016/j.ogc.2022.02.011.

## REFERENCES

1. Moore JF, Carugno J. Hysteroscopy. [Updated 2021 Dec 5]. In: StatPearls [Internet]. Treasure Island (FL): StatPearls Publishing; 2022 Jan. Available from: https://www.ncbi.nlm.nih.gov/books/NBK564345/.
2. Centini G, Troia L, Lazzeri L, et al. Modern operative hysteroscopy. Minerva Ginecol 2016;68(2):126–32.

3. Brooks PG. the management of abnormal uterine bleeding, is office hysteroscopy preferable to sonography? The case for hysteroscopy. J Minim Invasive Gynecol 2007;14(1):12–4.
4. Wortman M. See-and-Treat" hysteroscopy in the management of endometrial polyps. Surg Technol Int 2016;28:177–84.
5. Kelekci S, Kaya E, Alan M, et al. Comparison of transvaginal sonography, saline infusion sonography, and office hysteroscopy in reproductive-aged women with or without abnormal uterine bleeding. Fertil Steril 2005;84(3):682–6.
6. Yen CF, Chou HH, Wu HM, et al. Effectiveness and appropriateness in the application of office hysteroscopy. J Formos Med Assoc 2019;118(11):1480–7.
7. ACOG Committee Opinion No. 800. The use of hysteroscopy for the diagnosis and treatment of intrauterine pathology. Obstet Gynecol 2020;135:e138–48. Available at. https://www.acog.org/clinical/clinical-guidance/committee-opinion/articles/2020/03/the-use-of-hysteroscopy-for-the-diagnosis-and-treatment-of-intrauterine-pathology.
8. Robinson JK, Swedarsky LM, Colimon, et al. Postoperative adhesiolysis therapy for intrauterine adhesions (Asherman's syndrome). Fertil Steril 2008;90(2):409–14.
9. Salazar CA, Isaacson KB. Office operative hysteroscopy: an update. J Minim Invasive Gynecol 2018;25(2):199–208.
10. Wright KN, Simko S. Getting started with office hysteroscopy. Contemp OB/GYN J 2021;66(9):28–32.
11. Gambadauro P, Martínez-Maestre MA, Torrejón R. When is see-and-treat hysteroscopic polypectomy successful? Eur J Obstet Gynecol Reprod Biol 2014;178:70–3.
12. Marsh FA, Rogerson LJ, Duffy SR. A randomised controlled trial comparing outpatient versus daycase endometrial polypectomy. BJOG 2006;113(8):896–901.
13. ACOG Committee on Practice Bulletins–Gynecology. ACOG practice bulletin no. 104: antibiotic prophylaxis for gynecologic procedures. Obstet Gynecol 2009;113(5):1180–9.
14. Vitale SG, Bruni S, Chiofalo B, et al. Updates in office hysteroscopy: a practical decalogue to perform a correct procedure. Updates Surg 2020;72(4):967–76.
15. Munro MG, Storz K, et al. AAGL practice report: practice guidelines for the management of hysteroscopic distending media. J Minim Invasive Gynecol 2013;20(2):137–48. Available at. https://www.aagl.org/wp-content/uploads/2013/03/aagl-Practice-Guidelines-for-the-Management-of-Hysteroscopic-Distending-Media.pdf.
16. Emanuel MH. New developments in hysteroscopy. Best Pract Res Clin Obstet Gynaecol 2013;27(3):421–9.
17. Marty R. Decontamination, disinfection and sterilization of the hysteroscopes. In: Office and operative hysteroscopy. Paris: Springer; 2002. https://doi.org/10.1007/978-2-8178-0841-3_6. Available at.
18. TruClear system elite hysteroscopes cleaning and sterilization guide. Medtronic 2020. Available at. https://asiapac.medtronic.com/content/dam/covidien/library/us/en/product/gynecology-products/truclear-system-elite-hysteroscope-sterilization-guide.pdf. Downloaded on Oct 13, 2021.
19. CIDEX OPA solution. Product page from advanced sterilization products. Available at: https://www.asp.com/products/high-level-disinfection/cidex-opa-solution.

20. Prolystica® Surgical Instrument Cleaning Chemistries. Product page from STE-RIS Healthcare. Available at: https://www.steris.com/healthcare/products/surgical-instrument-cleaning-chemistries/prolystica-surgical-instrument-cleaning-chemistries.
21. Angioli R, De Cicco Nardone C, Plotti F, et al. Use of music to reduce anxiety during office hysteroscopy: prospective randomized trial. J Minim Invasive Gynecol 2014;21(3):454–9.
22. Gambadauro P, Navaratnarajah R, Carli V. Anxiety at outpatient hysteroscopy. Gynecol Surg 2015;12(3):189–96.
23. Bettocchi S, Ceci O, Di Venere R, et al. Advanced operative office hysteroscopy without anaesthesia: analysis of 501 cases treated with a 5 Fr. bipolar electrode. Hum Reprod 2002;17(9):2435–8.
24. Cicinelli E. Hysteroscopy without anesthesia: review of recent literature. J Minim Invasive Gynecol 2010;17(6):703–8.
25. De Silva PM, Mahmud A, Smith PP, et al. Analgesia for office hysteroscopy: a systematic review and meta-analysis. J Minim Invasive Gynecol 2020;27(5):1034–47.
26. Brunn E, Cheney M, Hazen N, Robinson JK. Virtual reality effects on acute pain during office hysteroscopy: a randomized control trial. J Gyncol Surg 2022. https://doi.org/10.1089/gyn.2021.0121.
27. Hua Y, Zhang W, Hu X, et al. The use of misoprostol for cervical priming prior to hysteroscopy: a systematic review and analysis. Drug Des Devel Ther 2016;10:2789–801.
28. Penketh RJ, Bruen EM, White J, et al. Feasibility of resectoscopic operative hysteroscopy in a UK outpatient clinic using local anesthetic and traditional reusable equipment, with patient experiences and comparative cost analysis. J Minim Invasive Gynecol 2014;21(5):830–6.
29. Bennett A, Lepage C, Thavorn K, et al. Effectiveness of outpatient versus operating room hysteroscopy for the diagnosis and treatment of uterine conditions: a systematic review and meta-analysis. J Obstet Gynaecol Can 2019;41(7):930–41.

# Hysteroscopic Myomectomy

Nash S. Moawad, MD, MS[a],*, Hannah Palin, MD[b]

## KEYWORDS

• Fibroids • Submucosal • Hysteroscopic myomectomy

## KEY POINTS

• Uterine fibroids are very common, and some are symptomatic.
• There is a wide spectrum of fibroids in terms of location, number, size, and symptomatology.
• Asymptomatic fibroids can be managed expectantly.
• Submucosal fibroids are implicated in abnormal uterine bleeding and subfertility.
• Hysteroscopic myomectomy is the treatment of choice for symptomatic submucosal myomas.

 Video content accompanies this article at http://www.obgyn.theclinics.com.

## INTRODUCTION

Hysteroscopy is an essential tool in every gynecologic practice offering minimally invasive evaluation and treatment for intrauterine pathology. Technology used in hysteroscopic procedures has improved steadily throughout the last two decades with improvements in optics, fluid management systems, and instrumentation for removal of intrauterine pathology. Pathology that once might have required an arduous and lengthy hospital procedure under general anesthesia can now be treated in minutes in an office setting. Similarly, leiomyomas that would have required hysterectomy for treatment can now be easily and efficiently resected in the operating room. These advancements have enabled a paradigm shift to the consideration of hysteroscopy for all patients with suspected endometrial pathology. It has also allowed the transition of many hysteroscopic procedures to the office setting. Advances in technology have allowed for faster operating times and more complete treatment of intrauterine pathology. Simultaneously, the efficiency and the safety of uterine cavity evaluation and

[a] Division of Minimally Invasive Gynecologic Surgery, Department of Obstetrics & Gynecology, University of Florida College of Medicine, PO Box 100294, Gainesville, FL 32610, USA; [b] Minimally Invasive Gynecologic Surgery, Mayo Clinic, 4500 San Pablo Road South, Jacksonville, FL 32224, USA
* Corresponding author.
*E-mail address:* nmoawad@ufl.edu
Twitter: @NMoawad_MIGS (N.S.M.)

Obstet Gynecol Clin N Am 49 (2022) 329–353
https://doi.org/10.1016/j.ogc.2022.02.012
0889-8545/22/Published by Elsevier Inc.

obgyn.theclinics.com

treatment provide patients with faster recovery and return to normal activities. With the hysteroscopic evaluation of the uterine cavity, the role of blind biopsies, dilation and curettage, and polypectomy is becoming increasingly questionable.[1] This article seeks to provide an in-depth and up-to-date exploration of hysteroscopic myomectomy, with a concise review of the pathology, clinical presentation, and the preoperative and postoperative management.

## LEIOMYOMAS

Uterine leiomyomas arise from the smooth muscle cells and fibroblasts of the myometrium, although the exact inciting factor for growth is not known. Upregulation of steroid receptors can also increase growth factors and mitogenic factors that recruit surrounding immature cells and growing leiomyoma tissue.[2,3] Aromatase activity has also been found to be 2 to 20 fold higher in leiomyoma tissues than in smooth muscle cells in culture.[4] The propagating cells, therefore, create their own hormone-driven environment.

Estrogen has long been thought to be the primary cause of fibroid growth. Estrogen receptors are more prolific in the tissue of leiomyomata when compared with normal myometrial tissue. Nuclear estrogen receptors are made from 2 similar genes forming either alpha or beta receptors (ER $\alpha$ or ER $\beta$). Patients who had a solitary leiomyoma were found to have higher levels of ER $\alpha$, whereas those with multiple leiomyomas had higher levels of ER $\beta$.[5] Other studies have pointed to a higher ratio of ER $\alpha$ to ER $\beta$ in attempting to describe the growth potential of myomas.[6] Regardless of the role of the specific receptor type, estradiol is certainly known to increase progesterone receptors, which increases tissue response to progesterone.[7] Progesterone is an important factor in the growth and proliferation of fibroids. Progesterone was found necessary for the maintenance of the size of uterine leiomyomas, and with its withdrawal, volume significantly decreased.[8]

In 2008, Peddada and colleagues reported on 72 women with a combined 262 leiomyomas who were followed for 12 months using MRI technology. Their study elucidated the variances not just between patients but between each leiomyoma studied. On average, the growth rate of leiomyomas was 9% over 6 months but each tumor grew at a different rate with some even regressing spontaneously. The growth rate was not affected by tumor size or location; however, patients with solitary leiomyomas were found to have faster growth rates than those who had multiple leiomyomas.[9]

## EPIDEMIOLOGY

The symptoms of leiomyomas are linked to a patient's reproductive years as this is the time that hormones are consistent and active. Approximately half of women will have a uterine fibroid at some point in their life. Fibroids are the most common pelvic tumor diagnosed in women. It is difficult to understand the exact prevalence of fibroids as many patients are asymptomatic. One study found leiomyomas on histopathology in 77 of 100 uteri after hysterectomy and numerous fibroids were found in 84% of those specimens underlining the commonality of this diagnosis.[10]

There is an increased incidence of leiomyomas in Black women compared with Caucasian women. Studies of gene expression in leiomyoma tissue found that there were higher levels of aromatase mRNA in the leiomyoma tissue of African American women.[11] The rate of growth and the likelihood of rapid expansion of a fibroid decrease with age in Caucasian women, whereas the same does not occur in African American women.[9]

Patients who are obese, have increased alcohol intake, increased soybean milk consumption, a diet high in red meat, or have vitamin D deficiency are at greater risk.[12,13] Patients with high blood pressure also have a greater predilection to leiomyoma growth.[14] Lastly, there are genetic linkages believed to be associated with leiomyomas. Family history is a risk factor for uterine fibroids.[15] A genome-wide SNP linkage panel was created and analyzed 261 sister pairs finding linkages that reached genome-wide significance.[16] However, much work is needed to better understand and categorize this potential genetic predisposition.

## SYMPTOMATOLOGY

Fibroids can frequently be asymptomatic or incidentally diagnosed. Asymptomatic women should be educated about the benign nature of these tumors and reassured about their clinical course. A review of concerning symptoms and reasons to present to a health care setting can help to alleviate patients' anxiety and avoid unnecessary interventions.

For symptomatic women, approximately 70% of uterine fibroids manifest themselves with symptoms of abnormal uterine bleeding (AUB). This is the most common indication for hysteroscopic myomectomy. Submucosal fibroids are associated with AUB in an estimated 5% to 10% of cases,[17] plausibly secondary to distortion of the endometrial cavity leading to greater endometrial surface area and inability of the uterine musculature to adequately contract and tamponade the spiral arteries providing blood to the endometrium.[18] Other conjectures involve dysregulation of angiogenic factors such as vascular endothelial growth factor, platelet-derived growth factor, and so forth.[19] Hysteroscopic resection of leiomyomas has been reported to achieve symptomatic relief rates of 70% to 99%.[20]

Aside from bleeding, reasons for resection of submucosal fibroids range from concerns about infertility to dysmenorrhea and pelvic pain. A thorough review of the literature attributes an estimated 1% to 2.4% of infertility cases to uterine leiomyomas when no other cause of infertility has been diagnosed.[21] Infertility issues caused by submucosal fibroids have not been borne out in the literature and it is not known if fibroids affect natural fertility.[22] Some limited studies have suggested that patients who are aged less than 40 years and have had infertility for fewer than 5 years might benefit more from myomectomy resection for infertility.[23] The American Society for Reproductive Medicine currently states that resection should take place for cavity-distorting myomas to improve pregnancy rates and decrease the risk of early pregnancy loss.[24]

Patients with subserosal or large pedunculated fibroids will often comment on pelvic pressure, constipation, or bladder irritability.

The Fibroid Growth Study published by Davis and colleagues in 2009 discovered that patients, regardless of the number and size of fibroids, equally chose surgical intervention for symptomatic fibroids.[25] Effective medical management options to mitigate the pain and heavy bleeding episodes would likely lead to a decreased need for surgical intervention.

## CLASSIFICATIONS OF FIBROIDS

Several classifications have been proposed for uterine leiomyomas. In 2011, the FIGO classification of uterine leiomyomas (**Fig. 1**) has been introduced and has since been widely accepted and used to understand symptomatology as well as for surgical planning. Gynecologists have used FIGO types 1 to 8 to discuss surgical approaches and outcomes for abdominal and hysteroscopic procedures.[26,27] Hysteroscopic

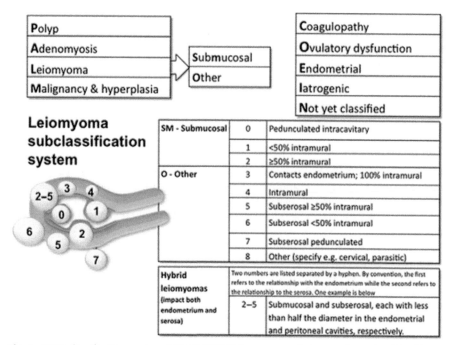

Fig. 1. FIGO classification system (PALM-COEIN) for causes of abnormal uterine bleeding in nongravid women of reproductive age. (*From* Munro MG, Critchley HO, Broder MS, Fraser IS; FIGO Working Group on Menstrual Disorders. FIGO classification system (PALM-COEIN) for causes of abnormal uterine bleeding in nongravid women of reproductive age. Int J Gynaecol Obstet. 2011;113(1):3-13. https://doi.org/10.1016/j.ijgo.2010.11.011; with permission.)

myomectomy is typically confined to FIGO type 0 through type 2, and occasionally type 3 (**Fig. 2**).

### STEP-W Classification

Another classification system, developed in 2005 by Lasmar and colleagues (**Fig. 3**), used 5 parameters to classify submucosal fibroids to estimate the degree of difficulty of the hysteroscopic myomectomy.[28]

These 5 parameters included size, topography, extension of the base in relation to the uterine wall, penetration into the myometrium, and whether the fibroid is arising from the lateral wall (STEP-W). In a study of 62 hysteroscopic myomectomies, Lasmar and colleagues showed that the STEP-W classification had a good correlation with surgical difficulty. A follow-up multicenter study in 2011 with 465 myomectomies again showed a good correlation of the STEP-W classification with complete or incomplete removal of the fibroid at the time of hysteroscopic myomectomy.[29]

### IMAGING

Appropriate evaluation of the location and number of uterine fibroids is crucial for the evaluation of patient complaints, counseling, options for treatment, and surgical planning.

Imaging almost universally begins with transvaginal ultrasound. Pelvic ultrasound has excellent sensitivity for diagnosing fibroids with limitations increasing if the

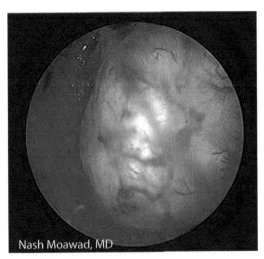

**Fig. 2.** Type 1 submucosal fibroid.

patient is pregnant, if there are multiple fibroids, or if the patient cannot tolerate transvaginal ultrasound.[30] If diagnostic hysteroscopy is readily available in the office, many physicians will use hysteroscopy to complement ultrasound findings. Some gynecologists argue for evaluation with saline infusion sonography (SIS) for proper evaluation of the fibroid and its relationship to the uterine cavity. When findings from transvaginal ultrasound are inconclusive about the type of fibroid found, the addition of SIS is a good second-line diagnostic procedure.[31] Both procedures are found to be effective in diagnosing intracavitary fibroids with excellent agreement (92%) between modalities in the case of types 0 1 fibroids.[30,32] MRI is also frequently used for preoperative workup and surgical planning, particularly for larger

|   | Size (cm) | Topography | Extension of the base | Penetration | Lateral Wall | Total |
|---|---|---|---|---|---|---|
| 0 | >2 to 5 | Low | ≤1/3 | 0 | | |
| 1 | >2 to 5 | Middle | >1/3 to 2/3 | ≤50% | **+1** | |
| 2 | >5 | Upper | >2/3 | >50% | | |
| Score | + | + | + | + | + | |

| Score | Group | Complexity and therapeutic options |
|---|---|---|
| 0 to 4 | I | Low complexity hysteroscopic myomectomy. |
| 5 to 6 | II | High complexity hysteroscopic myomectomy. Consider GnRH use? Consider Two-step hysteroscopic myomectomy. |
| 7 to 9 | III | Consider alternatives to the hysteroscopic technique |

**Fig. 3.** LASMAR/STEP-W Classification for submucosal leiomyomas and prediction of surgical difficulty. (*From* Lasmar RB, Lasmar BP, Celeste RK, da Rosa DB, Depes Dde B, Lopes RG. A new system to classify submucous myomas: a Brazilian multicenter study. J Minim Invasive Gynecol. 2012;19(5):575-580. https://doi.org/10.1016/j.jmig.2012.03.026; with permission.)

and multiple fibroids requiring laparoscopic or robot-assisted myomectomy. A randomized control trial (RCT) of 18 women undergoing ultrasound and MRI showed that MRI had superior sensitivity with better correlation to the actual size of pathology over transvaginal ultrasound.[33] However, patient characteristics such as sexual activity, pelvic pain, and anxiety levels should also be considered when ordering imaging for the evaluation of fibroids. Patients were found to have higher levels of fear, anxiety, and mental and physical issues after MRI versus TVUS but greater embarrassment during TVUS.[34]

It is important to also note the role that ultrasound imaging can play for the practitioner in cases of difficult hysteroscopy or concern for transmural leiomyomas requiring resection.[35] Ultrasound-guidance has been used in the operating room with great success and should be considered for patients with distorted anatomy or difficult entry into the uterus.

## PREOPERATIVE ASSESSMENT

Patient selection is an important part of all surgical workup. Abnormal bleeding and bulk or pressure symptoms are some of the most common symptoms prompting women to seek care for large uterine fibroids. Patients who are undergoing fertility workup and have a submucosal fibroid are also appropriate candidates for surgical management. Regardless of the surgical approach of myomectomy, patients have improved quality of life scores and decreased symptom severity.[36] This article focuses on surgical management with hysteroscopic myomectomy.

To ensure appropriate shared decision making with patients, all feasible treatment options should be discussed with each patient, including expectant management. Medical management should be the first line when available and appropriate for the patient's symptoms and goals. The patient's comorbid conditions and prior surgical history should be obtained and can help to guide counseling. Lack of desire for future fertility, suspicion of concomitant uterine pathology, or failed prior myomectomy are some examples to consider more definitive surgical management with hysterectomy. Some patients prefer the most conservative approach possible, whereas others may find the potential for regrowth of fibroids and reintervention unacceptable. If future fertility is a consideration, it is important to address the patient's concerns, ensure proper counseling, and engage in consultation with a reproductive endocrinologist as needed before finalizing surgical treatment plans. When patients feel confident in their decision for a particular procedure before surgical intervention, higher patient satisfaction scores result postoperatively.[37] This challenges providers to ensure that they are individualizing patient counseing instead of making broad recommendations based on age or other demographic factors.

A proper physical examination is also necessary and important for many reasons. Providers should ensure that there are no other obvious causes for AUB. Vaginal atrophy should be addressed and gross lesions on the cervix should be properly evaluated. The physical examination should also ensure that there are no prolapsing fibroids or cervical polyps that could cause symptoms of pain or AUB. During the physical examination, the physician should note whether the patient can tolerate speculum examination well and could potentially tolerate an in-office procedure for further workup before surgery or even potentially undergo hysteroscopic management in the office. We also recommend noting whether there is a need to dilate or open the cervix for procedures to be properly prepared with lacrimal duct dilators or scalpel for cruciate incision of the cervix, or for hysteroscopic dilation of the cervix during vaginoscopy. After the physical examination is performed, proper laboratory assessment and imaging should be subsequently ordered.

Patients with heavy bleeding and concern for anemia should have a complete blood count drawn and proper intervention in the case of severe anemia. If there is concern for mass effect on the bladder or ureters, it is appropriate to order a basic metabolic panel to evaluate kidney function and consider imaging the kidneys and ureters. A pregnancy test should be performed for all reproductive-age women before surgical management. Lastly, those patients who desire future fertility and are undergoing surgery for that sole purpose should be evaluated by a reproductive endocrinologist and determination should be made about their reproductive health and options.

## OFFICE HYSTEROSCOPY

Given the advances in technology previously mentioned, office hysteroscopy is more affordable and easier to perform than ever before. Preoperative planning with office hysteroscopy is feasible for surgical planning and appropriate patient counseling. Small, 1 to 2 cm type 0 submucosal myomas can potentially be removed in the office setting using hysteroscopic scissors or tissue removal systems. A prospective study of patient outcomes after hysteroscopic myomectomy found higher successful completion rates when the fibroids were ≤3 cm in size.[38] However, this was for all hysteroscopies and even this size may be difficult for patients undergoing an office procedure. Incision of the pseudocapsule during office hysteroscopy may allow the protrusion of the fibroid into the uterine cavity, improving the likelihood of complete resection during subsequent hysteroscopic myomectomy.[39] The advent of the miniresectoscope and the tissue removal devices has improved our ability to remove larger submucosal fibroids in the office setting.

## PHARMACOLOGIC INTERVENTION AND PREOPERATIVE PATIENT OPTIMIZATION
### Oral and Intravenous Iron Supplementation

Anemia is defined as a hemoglobin level of less than 120 g/L for women. Iron deficiency anemia secondary to chronic blood loss can be treated in numerous ways including blood transfusion, oral iron supplementation, or intravenous (IV) iron infusion. However, blood transfusion is not considered a first-line option, given its risk profile and associated complications and cost. In patients who are undergoing elective surgery without active bleeding and symptomatic anemia, it is preferable to supplement with iron.

Oral iron is a good first-line treatment if patients can tolerate it. There are known gastrointestinal side effects and if the patient has other concomitant issues with malabsorption (Inflammatory Bowel Disease or malignancy), then it can decrease the efficacy of oral treatment. Approximately 70% of patients complain of reflux, constipation, and/or abdominal pain when taking oral supplementation. Various preparations of iron exist, all of which are available over the counter. Recent developments of new ferric compounds and ferrous salts have improved symptomatology and are "not affected by food, milk or medicines which permits its ingestion during or after meals and the tolerability... is much better."[40] It takes approximately 1 to 2 months for the treatment of iron deficiency anemia and another 3 to 6 months to replenish iron stores. If the patient continues to have bleeding throughout that time, this slow method of repletion might be ineffective for the patient.

IV iron is another option for patients with known iron deficiency anemia; IV supplementation works faster with a more substantial increase in hemoglobin levels than its oral counterpart. When initially introduced in the 1930s, iron preparations caused occasional anaphylactic responses. With the introduction of low-molecular-weight iron and reconfigured complexes, there is no longer a need for test dosing and doses as high as 1 g of iron can be given in a single administration.[41] This is excellent news for many patients who previously might have been at higher risk of blood transfusion without rapid correction of hemoglobin levels.

### Misoprostol

Preoperative preparation with misoprostol has been adopted into practice by many physicians to decrease bleeding during surgery. Its use has been established for open and laparoscopic myomectomies.[42] A meta-analysis of misoprostol use before myomectomy showed a statistically significant decrease in blood loss of 0.68 g/dL without significant side effects.[43] However, extrapolating that data to hysteroscopic myomectomy has yet to lead to any definitive conclusions about blood loss. Misoprostol in assisting with cervical dilation can be helpful for patients in whom entry into the uterine cavity might be difficult. However, the softening of the cervix can also lead to overdilation and fluid loss during the procedure. Decisions to use misoprostol should be individualized.[44]

### Ulipristal Acetate

Ulipristal acetate (a selective progesterone receptor modulator) has also been studied for potential use before surgical intervention on intrauterine fibroids. Preoperative treatment for 3 to 6 months before intervention increased the percentage of completely resected type 0 to 1 fibroids compared with patients who went immediately to surgery (89%–68.9%).[45] Another study determined that its use before hysteroscopic management did not negatively affect surgical outcomes but more data are needed to determine its clinical utility.[46]

### GnRH Agonist

The use of GnRH agonists in preparation for hysteroscopic myomectomy is limited to the treatment of baseline anemia in preparation for surgery, and to potentially decrease the size of submucosal fibroids if it will facilitate the procedure and improve the likelihood of complete removal of the fibroid. In patients in whom heavy menstrual bleeding is causing significant anemia, pretreatment with GnRH agonists can stop bleeding for long enough to improve hemoglobin levels before surgery[47] There is suggestion that the greatest benefit may be in pretreatment with GnRH agonist therapy before hysteroscopic resection. GnRH agonist treatment causes endometrial atrophy, which assists with hysteroscopic visualization, thereby decreasing operative time. Studies have also shown decreased fluid absorption during hysteroscopy in pretreated uteri. Lower fluid absorption levels decrease the risks during prolonged resection for a large submucosal fibroid. One study showed improvement in complete fibroid resection with the use of GnRH agonist treatment before hysteroscopic myomectomy when compared with controls (3% vs 20%),[48] though others have not found the same improvement when performing cold loop resection.[49] A randomized, multicenter study showed decreased operative times and decreased fluid absorption when a GnRH analogue was used before hysteroscopic resection of submucosal fibroids.[50] A small study of 25 patients also evaluated and found benefit in pretreatment for hysteroscopic myomectomy in patients who were considered inoperative because of leiomyoma size.[51] Certainly, more research is needed to understand the utility before hysteroscopic procedures.

## HYSTEROSCOPIC MYOMECTOMY—THE PROCEDURE
### Optimization

#### Paracervical blocks

There is conflicting evidence about paracervical blocks and their efficacy in outpatient procedures. It has been studied more thoroughly in the Family Planning literature for use during surgical procedures requiring dilation of the cervix. This form of anesthesia has been proven effective in other procedures including second-trimester laminaria placement and intrauterine device placement.[52] Its use compared to other forms of pain management in operative hysteroscopy has not been shown to be superior in many studies.[53] A Cochrane Database review which included 26 studies on the utility of paracervical block did not conclusively determine whether paracervical injection of local anesthetic made any difference. It was not found to be superior, but 10 studies compared paracervical block with placebo and found a decreased risk of severe pain (RR 0.16) and reduced pain on cervical dilation and during the time of uterine intervention. There was no evidence to infer its superiority to other pain management options.[54] Only 55% of women would recommend this form of analgesia after undergoing a procedure with paracervical block.[55] Given that its efficacy cannot be proven regarding hysteroscopy but has been found to be beneficial with other forms of cervical and uterine manipulation, this form of analgesia should be used as an additional tool at the physician's discretion after proper patient counseling.

    Normal dosing of lidocaine is shown in the following table. Dosing varies depending on the type of analgesic used and whether it is mixed with epinephrine. It is important to recall the side effects of toxicity. First, the patient's lips or tongue will become numb, which prompts patients to complain of "tingling lips" or slurred speech. Next, cardiovascular effects, such as hypotension, bradycardia, or arrhythmias, can occur. Muscle twitching or tremors and seizures can then occur and finally respiratory depression and cardiac arrest. Patients should be properly informed of the side effects of lidocaine toxicity and encouraged to report side effects immediately to avoid severe complications.

| | Dosage | Maximum Dosage Without Epinephrine | Maximum Dosage With Epinephrine |
|---|---|---|---|
| Lidocaine | 1% = 10 mg/mL 2% = 20 mg/mL | 5 mg/kg | 7 mg/kg |

#### Vasopressin

Vasopressin has long been used in laparoscopy and open cases to decrease blood flow to fibroids during myomectomy, thereby decreasing surgical blood loss and potentially improving visualization, maximizing efficiency, and decreasing the risk of complications. During hysteroscopy, vasopressin can be injected directly into the myoma using a cystoscopic needle through the operative channel under hysteroscopic guidance. A prospective, double-blind RCT of 40 women found that there was a statistically significant improvement in the surgical field, decreased operative blood loss, and decreased fluid intravasation. However, this did not translate to reduced operative time.[56] Another option is to inject vasopressin into the cervical stroma. This has been associated with decreased fluid intravasation, decreased blood loss, and decreased operative time.

    Current recommendations call for 10 units of vasopressin in 100 to 200 mL of normal saline, which is injected in small aliquots with care being taken to avoid any intravascular injection. There is no consensus on the limit of vasopressin that should be used in a procedure but a maximum of 4 to 6 units has been proposed.[57] Repeat dosing can be performed at approximately 45 minutes duration if bleeding increases. The full duration of action of vasopressin is believed to be 2 to 8 hours. Intravascular injection or overinjection has been associated with cardiovascular complications such as severe bradycardia, hypertension, and even death. Judicious use is imperative in patients with prior cardiovascular issues or significant renal disease.

### Fluid Management and Distension Media

Contemporary hysteroscopic surgery has evolved to use 1 of 2 fluid distending media; electrolyte-rich or electrolyte-poor depending on the type of energy used for the procedure. Electrolyte-poor solutions such as 5% dextrose, 1.5% glycine, 3% sorbitol, or 5% mannitol must be used with monopolar energy to allow for monopolar current to be effectively focused and prevent it from getting dispersed throughout the uterus. Electrolyte-rich solutions include normal saline and lactated Ringer solutions, which are used in conjunction with bipolar energy.

Recommendations are made to use an intrauterine pressure of 70 to 80 mm Hg, which is approximately equal to the mean arterial pressure for the average patient. The goal is to decrease the risk of intravasation due to higher pressures. If visualization is decreased because of bleeding or large pathology and higher pressures are necessary, the pressure may be increased for a short period to achieve adequate visualization and facilitate completion of the procedure.

There are various ways to instill fluid in a hysteroscopic procedure, including gravity for fluid pressure with each increase in height of 0.3 m increasing the fluid pressure by 25 mm Hg. This can be assisted by a pressure bag that continues flow to the hysteroscopic system even with low levels of fluid. We recommend the use of automated systems for most operative hysteroscopies, given their ease of use and delivery of constant pressure and continuous flow of the distension media.

It is important to monitor the "fluid deficit" for patients during each procedure. There are many automated systems now in use that automatically account for the input and output of fluid. If there is significant bleeding during the procedure, this should also be acknowledged as it can artificially increase the amount of return and underestimate the fluid deficit. There are also reports of incorrectly filled fluid bags that can be as much as 6% higher than the 3L stated on the bags.[58] These limitations make it favorable to use an automated system when available.

### The Technology

Hysteroscopic myomectomy is the conservative minimally invasive procedure used to definitively resect submucosal fibroids. Its low-risk profile and excellent outcomes make it a mainstay of treatment for symptomatic submucosal fibroids.[59] There are numerous technologies that can be used with the goal of removing the fibroid in its entirety whether it is a G0, G1, or G2 type fibroid. There is a plethora of hysteroscopic devices used for resection of leiomyoma, which are reviewed in the following sections.

#### Wire loop resectoscope

The wire loop resectoscope is a commonly used instrument in a hysteroscopic myomectomy, using an operative hysteroscope (Resectoscope) (**Figs. 4–6**). Ideally, a 12° scope would be used to keep the tip of the wire loop in view throughout the entire procedure. Use of a 0° scope limits visualization. The resectoscope can be used with either monopolar or bipolar current. A study looking at monopolar versus bipolar electrosurgery looked at side effects after hysteroscopy. It was noted that bipolar

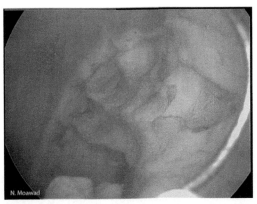

**Fig. 4.** Bipolar loop electrode used for hysteroscopic myomectomy of large type 1 submucosal myoma.

electrosurgery had a better safety profile because of the use of isotonic solution to distend the endometrial cavity. It is critical to use the correct distention medium when using the electrosurgery as discussed previously in this chapter. The monopolar device requires an electrolyte-poor solution, which was found to cause significant electrolyte disturbance in this study. Patients' serum sodium levels dropped by approximately 5 mmol/L (138.7 mmol/L to 133.8 mmol/L).[60] Monopolar devices are also known to cause higher thermal spread because of their low-frequency current, which penetrates further into the tissue and spreads further from the point of contact. This can inadvertently lead to thermal damage of the surrounding endometrium and myometrium during dissection. Bipolar current remains between the electrodes of the device and is found to have a depth of penetration of less than 1 mm as compared with 3 to 5 mm with monopolar systems.[61] The loop electrode is used to resect tissue starting at the cephalad portion of the myoma and moving caudad, shaving off pieces with electrosurgery while maintaining hemostasis. This movement prevents the unnecessary risk of perforation that can occur with a forward caudad to cephalad motion. Bipolar devices have higher coagulation capacities, which prevents the need for repeated coagulation during a procedure due to bleeding. It is important to continue the resection to include the intramural portion of the submucosal fibroid, after separating it within the pseudocapsule plane. Manipulating the intrauterine pressure is

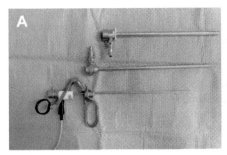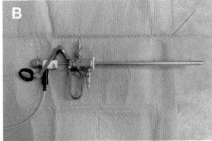

**Fig. 5.** (A) Resectoscope with bipolar cord attached, inflow and outflow channels shown in ascending order. (B) Resectoscope with bipolar cord attached, inflow and outflow channels attached.

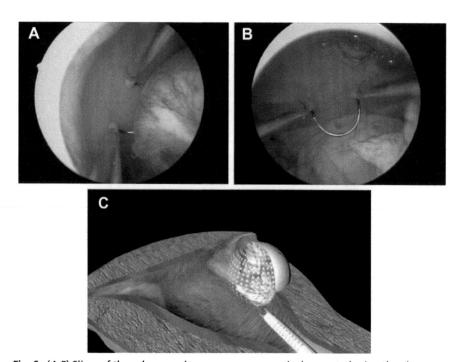

**Fig. 6.** (*A,B*) Slices of the submucosal myoma are progressively resected using the electrosurgical loop. (*C*) The Cold Loop technique is used to bluntly dissect the fibroid from the surrounding myometrium in the pseudocapsule plain. (*From* Mazzon I, Favilli A, Grasso M, Horvath S, Di Renzo GC, Gerli S. Is Cold Loop Hysteroscopic Myomectomy a Safe and Effective Technique for the Treatment of Submucous Myomas With Intramural Development? A Series of 1434 Surgical Procedures. J Minim Invasive Gynecol. 2015;22(5):792-798. https://doi.org/10.1016/j.jmig.2015.03.004; with permission.)

important to allow the fibroid to protrude further into the uterine cavity and facilitate complete resection. The procedure is limited by the maximum allowable fluid deficit. As discussed previously, a higher fluid deficit with isotonic electrolyte solution is permissible compared with an electrolyte-poor solution, which causes greater serum electrolyte disturbances. Once the predetermined deficit is reached, the procedure should be concluded, and a staged procedure can be considered later if needed.

### Cold loop dissection
Cold loop dissection (**Fig. 7**) is another option for removal of submucosal fibroids that is advocated for because of its low-risk profile and its respect for tissue integrity, by taking advantage of the pseudocapsule and using this plane for blunt dissection. This technique is considered optimal for fibroids with an intramural component because of its safety profile and decreased risk to surrounding tissue. First introduced by Mazzon in 1995,[62] this technique can be combined with the resectoscopic technique to achieve complete removal of the deeper portions of types 1 and 2 submucosal myomas.[63] The same resectoscope that was described earlier is used with a few additional steps. The technique begins with normal dissection of the intramural component of the fibroid with monopolar or bipolar electrocautery. When the level of the endometrium is reached, it is critical to stop dissecting the fibroid tissue with electrocautery. The next step is to find and develop the plane between the myoma

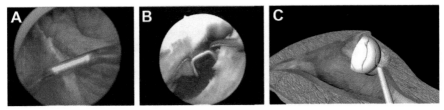

Fig. 7. (*A*) The electric cutting loop is subsequently replaced with a cold loop, which is inserted into the cleavage plane and repeatedly applied along the surface of the myoma. (*B*, *C*) Then the cold loop is used to detach the fibroconnective bridges that anchor the myoma to the pseudocapsule. (*From* Mazzon I, Favilli A, Grasso M, Horvath S, Di Renzo GC, Gerli S. Is Cold Loop Hysteroscopic Myomectomy a Safe and Effective Technique for the Treatment of Submucous Myomas With Intramural Development? A Series of 1434 Surgical Procedures. J Minim Invasive Gynecol. 2015;22(5):792-798. https://doi.org/10.1016/j.jmig. 2015.03.004; with permission.)

and the myometrium. There are various cold loop attachments that can then be used to bluntly dissect the connective tissue that anchors the fibroid to the surrounding myometrium. As more of the myoma enters the cavity after separation from the surrounding tissue, it can be removed using electrocautery if desired. A large retrospective review of 1215 patients showed a completion rate of 83.7% with one surgical procedure. And importantly, the complication rate was 0.84% with no perforations in this cohort.[62]

For illustration of a combination of resectoscopic myomectomy and the cold loop technique, please refer to Video 1.

### Tissue extraction devices

Tissue extraction devices for hysteroscopic myomectomy work by using fragmentation and suction for simultaneous dissection and removal of tissue from the uterine cavity. There are various brands that have come on the market (eg, Myosure, Truclear, Symphion) and are mainly used for types 0 and 1 intrauterine leiomyomas (**Figs. 8** and **9**). A rotating blade incises the fibroid, and it is suctioned into a straining canister to separate the tissue from distension media for pathologic evaluation after the procedure. This technique alleviates the need for removal of fibroid "chips" from the cavity and it is easier for trainees to learn. A reusable 0° hysteroscope is coupled with a

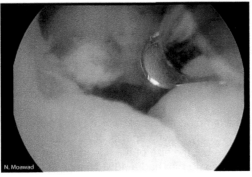

Fig. 8. Hysteroscopic tissue removal systems are the most recent advances in hysteroscopic myomectomy.

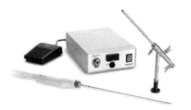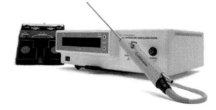

**Fig. 9.** Hysteroscopic tissue removal systems (*Left*: Myosure; *Right*: TruClear). (*From* Meulen-broeks D, Hamerlynck TW, Saglam-Kara S, Van Rijssel NK, Van Vliet HA, Schoot BC. Hysteroscopic Tissue Removal Systems: A Randomized In Vitro Comparison [published correction appears in J Minim Invasive Gynecol. 2017 Nov - Dec;24(7):1245]. J Minim Invasive Gynecol. 2017;24(1):159-164. https://doi.org/10.1016/j.jmig.2016.08.829; with permission).

single-use tissue extraction device that is inserted into an operative channel. These devices are disposable and require specific tubing to be connected to various fluid management systems. There are, however, limitations with these devices. First, the cost of the single-use elements is high and may be prohibitive to certain patients or in certain low-resource environments. It is also difficult to resect fundal fibroids as well as the deeper portions of types 1 and 2 fibroids with these devices. Lastly, some studies have found that dense myomas or those with calcifications can dull the rotating blades and make efficient or complete extraction difficult. One study showed that switching to a resectoscope in these cases allowed for finalization of the procedure.[64] However, another meta-analyses showed statistically significant improvement ($P = .002$) in complete resection of pathology when tissue extraction devices were used.[65] Depending on the size, makeup, and location of the fibroid, the surgeon should decide their preference for the type of device for submucosal fibroid resection.

**Comparison of device type.** As mentioned previously, the size, number, and type of the myomas encountered can affect the success rate of each procedure. A size greater than 3 cm is positively correlated with increased risk for need for multiple procedures.[38] A systematic review of hysteroscopic removal of submucosal fibroids reiterated that the classification of the fibroid is what is most related to the success rate for complete removal. Types 0 and 1 have a higher likelihood of complete resection than type 2.[66] In another cohort study, the size of myomas resected was also directly correlated with the likelihood of success for completion in a single-step procedure (OR 1.052). The larger the myoma, the more likely it would need to be performed in a multi-step procedure.[67] The same study found that a type 0 fibroid had a 100% chance of resection in a single-step procedure, whereas the likelihood of removing a type 2 fibroid in a single-step procedure decreased to 82.55%. A systematic review of hysteroscopic removal of submucosal fibroids reiterated that the classification of the fibroid is what is most related to the success rate for complete removal. Types 0 and 1 have a higher likelihood of complete resection than type 2.[66] There is no doubt that the characteristics of the myoma will determine the probability of successful completion.

Some studies have attempted to discern which types of devices might have a high likelihood of success. A study looking specifically at tissue extraction devices found that it was not the device but the size of the fibroid that determined success. In that study, fibroids greater than 40 mm had a 48% chance of complete resection during an initial surgery and 10% of patients required further surgical intervention.[68] The efficacy of the resectoscope in removing submucosal fibroids shows mixed data. Litta and colleagues[69] noted a 100% rate of complete resection of types 1 and 2 with the bipolar resectoscope. Similarly, a review by Friedman and colleagues strongly stated that the strength of the resectoscope lies in its ability to tackle type 2 myomas.[70] A recently published study of 53 patients indicated that the newest iteration of the Myosure device completely resects type 2 fibroids in 96% of procedures.[71] The purported benefits of hysteroscopic tissue extraction devices lie in their improved visualization as this leads to shorter operative times.[72,73] However, there are critiques that these studies that look at operative times do not account for the difficulty in removal of type 2 myomas, which is more often undertaken with the resectoscope. Yet another review by each provider must choose their technique based on level of comfort with each device as well as size and type of fibroid encountered. An individualized approach to each patient and procedure is recommended.

## TECHNICAL TIPS AND TRICKS

It is important for the surgeon to choose the best tool for the pathology encountered. It is important to understand how each device is used and ensure proper setup. The surgeon must understand how to troubleshoot the hysteroscopic and resectoscopic devices, how to properly adjust and manage fluid media and intrauterine pressure, and how to quickly diagnose and treat complications such as fluid overload or embolism. Each procedure should be individualized depending on the intrauterine pathology. A perfect example is the combination of dissecting the pseudocapsule of a fibroid using the cold loop technique, even if using the regular monopolar and bipolar electrodes without energy and using the energy to resect the fibroid with energy as it protrudes into the uterine cavity. Merging these 2 modalities (cold loop and electrosurgical resection) facilitates complete resection of the deeper intramural portions of fibroids while minimizing thermal damage to the surrounding myometrium and decreasing the risk of uterine perforation. A large type 0 fibroid may be faster to approach using the tissue removal device, whereas a deeper type 1 or 2 fibroid, or a fundal fibroid, will lend itself better to resection using a combination of the wire loop resectoscope and the cold loop technique. Tactfully varying the intrauterine pressure periodically to allow the deeper portions of the fibroid, particularly types 2 and 3, to protrude into the uterine cavity, will facilitate the complete resection of these more challenging fibroids. The intrauterine pressure can be increased periodically to tamponade bleeding to avoid excessive use of energy and associated thermal damage. Withdrawal of the hysteroscope to remove fibroid chips and reinsertion of the hysteroscope should be kept to a minimum, to decrease the length of the procedure and the inevitable bleeding that ensues upon removal of the scope. Decreasing the number of times the scope is removed and reinserted increases efficiency and prevents delays caused by reestablishing visualization of the surgical field after removal of the device. Above all, the goal is to decrease severe morbidity including the rare, but catastrophic, air embolism that can be caused by the scope acting as piston forcing air/gas bubbles into the transected blood vessels.

## COMPLICATIONS
### Fluid Overload

As discussed earlier, fluid selection is an important part of the procedure itself. Fluid deficit limits were proposed as greater than 1000 mL of electrolyte-poor solution in a healthy, reproductive-age woman or 2500 mL deficit of isotonic, electrolyte-containing solution in a healthy, reproductive-age woman.[74] [75] Fluid overload, although rare, is a known complication of hysteroscopy that can become quite serious. It only occurs in up to 0.2% of cases but physicians performing this procedure should be comfortable with the symptoms of fluid overload as well as its prevention and basic management. Fluid overload is due to absorption of a high volume of fluid through intravasation, transtubal loss, and/or uterine perforation.[74] Risk factors for fluid overload are related to numerous patient factors as well as distention media used, intrauterine pressure, or prolonged operative times.

Patient factors include age and comorbid conditions. Young, healthy patients can tolerate a large amount of fluid absorption without issue. However, older patients or those with cardiopulmonary disorders, anemia, or renal dysfunction are at higher risk for complications. Volume overload, electrolyte abnormalities, and neurologic sequelae are the known side effects of excess fluid absorption. A patient's mean arterial pressure should be noted for these procedures. If the fluid distension pressure is higher than the patient's mean arterial pressure, fluid will more readily be absorbed into the vasculature. Most intrauterine surgery is now performed with saline distention media and bipolar energy, hence minimizing the risk of electrolyte imbalance and hyponatremia, but fluid overload is still a concern. Patients without comorbid conditions can tolerate up to 2500 mL of isotonic fluid deficit without sequelae. However, those with cardiac or pulmonary disorders can develop pulmonary edema and subsequent right heart strain due to excess fluid. Dependent on a patient's age, size, and other medical conditions, the limit of fluid deficit changes.

The type of distension medium used is also important to take into consideration when discussing the effects of overload. Electrolyte disturbances such as hyponatremia and hypo-osmolality should be taken into consideration. As discussed previously, with the use of monopolar electrocautery, it is necessary to use an electrolyte poor media such as glycine or sorbitol to prevent excitation of electrolytes with monopolar current. In the case of use of electrolyte poor fluid for distension, absorption can more readily cause electrolyte imbalance leading to neurologic sequelae. A decrease in serum tonicity forces increased flow of water across the blood-brain barrier, which causes the brain edema with symptoms being more pronounced depending on the abruptness of the change in tonicity.[76] Patients may show symptoms of fatigue, dizziness, gait disturbances, nausea and vomiting, muscle cramps and then confusion, and eventually lethargy and even mortality.[77]

The type of procedure performed also plays a role in fluid overload. When parts of the myometrium are resected, as in many operative hysteroscopy procedures, disrupted blood vessels are exposed to fluid under pressure, which increases intravascular absorption. Any procedure that may cause increased myometrial penetration will thereby increase absorption. Myomectomy carries greater risk because of the large blood vessels often found surrounding the leiomyomata. Larger fibroids also increase operative time, further prolonging the patient's exposure to fluid absorption. Lastly, the need to increase fluid pressure for better visualization can also lead to fluid overload as discussed with patient characteristics.

### Air Embolism

Air embolism can occur because of the use of gaseous media, gas introduced with fluid media, or creation of gas bubbles with vaporization during hysteroscopic electrosurgical procedures. Gas embolism can cause cardiovascular collapse and pulmonary edema. The classic "mill wheel" murmur is heard with acute changes in heart rate—either bradycardia or tachycardia. Acute management of gas embolism is out of the scope of this article but the anesthesia team caring for the patient should be quick to recognize signs of cardiovascular collapse to inform the surgical team of complications and treat quickly and efficiently.

Prevention of gas embolism is key and there are some important preventive steps that should be taken. The patient should never be placed in Trendelenburg position. During the priming process before initiation of a procedure, all air should be purged from the tubing before insertion into the uterus. This improves visualization and prevents the introduction of air bubbles into the uterine cavity. Pressure of less than 125 mm Hg should be used when possible to prevent forcing of gas into the vasculature. Insertion and removal of the devices used can also force gas into the cervix. Therefore, limiting the insertion and removal of the scope is also ideal as this is associated with increased risk of air or gas emboli.[78] In one study, gas embolism was significantly higher with a fluid deficit of greater than 1000 mL compared with less than 1000 mL.[79] Respecting fluid deficit limits can help to prevent gas embolism and not just fluid overload.

### Bleeding Complications

Significant life-threatening bleeding is rare with hysteroscopic myomectomy, but if encountered, balloon tamponade is recommended as a fast, safe, and cost-effective management tool.[80] As mentioned previously, the use of bipolar or monopolar electrosurgery can facilitate coagulation of encountered vasculature. Care must be taken to ensure appropriate depth of electrosurgery and to avoid excessive thermal spread.

### Perforation

Every patient should be counseled about the risks of possible perforation during hysteroscopy. Perforation is a rare complication of hysteroscopic myomectomy and is most commonly encountered at the time of cervical dilation. Cervical stenosis is a risk factor, such as in nulliparous or postmenopausal patients or patients with a history of cervical excisional procedure or cryotherapy. Perforation during the myomectomy is more common in cases of deep myomas involving the myometrium such as types 2 and 3 fibroids and is more common with fundal or cornual fibroids. If perforation using the activated resectoscope loop is encountered, laparoscopy should be performed because of the high risk of thermal damage to the bowel or bladder and the risk of bleeding.[80]

## CLINICAL OUTCOMES OF HYSTEROSCOPIC MYOMECTOMY
### Staged Procedures

Hysteroscopic procedures have improved in many ways as outlined in this article; however, there are some fibroids that still evade even the most advanced technology. As discussed earlier in detail, the classification of the fibroid plays a large role in determining the likelihood of complete resection with type 2 fibroids being the most difficult to remove. There are 2 classification systems that seek to preoperatively stratify myomas based on suspected level of surgical difficulty: STEP-W score (Lasmar's classification) and the ESGE classification (also with a Wamsteker modification).[81] [29] The STEP-W classification was previously mentioned and outlined in this article. New guidelines from the International Society for Gynecologic Endoscopy (ISGE) recommend using the STEP-W classification preoperatively to best counsel patients on the potential need for repeat surgical procedures and to assist surgeons in understanding suspected degree of difficulty.[82] This system uses several imaging characteristics to assess the degree of difficulty of hysteroscopic myomectomy and makes recommendations for treatment options. The goal with the utilization of these systems is to appropriately plan for procedures including the possibility of the need for 2-step procedures or even counseling against hysteroscopic myomectomy as a primary treatment choice.

When hysteroscopic myomectomy is complicated by fluid overload, patient intolerance, or concerns for other dangerous sequelae, they should immediately be terminated. However, if these concerns do not arise, then there are some techniques that can be attempted to prevent the need for repeat procedures due to incomplete resection. One such technique is called the multiple slicing sessions technique, where portions of the fibroid that are intrauterine are dissected to the level of the endometrium as usual. Next, a combination of "hydromassage," a technique that induces rapid changes in intrauterine pressure, and bimanual massage are used to stimulate uterine contractions forcing more of the fibroid into the uterine cavity for further resection.[83] In situations in which providers are concerned about the difficulty of the procedure, ultrasound guidance should be requested to facilitate safe removal.[84][85]

### Abnormal Uterine Bleeding

Multiple studies have reported a high success rate of 70% to 99% with hysteroscopic myomectomy. The rate depends on several variables, including the size, number and location of the fibroids, as well as the surgeon's expertise and whether resection was complete or incomplete. The rate of recurrent abnormal bleeding naturally increases with time, because of regrowth or recurrence of fibroids, incomplete removal, and the development of other etiologies for AUB.[80]

### Fertility outcomes

Submucosal leiomyomas are often implicated in the workup of patients with infertility. Hysteroscopic myomectomy is often discussed with patients as part of a grander treatment plan when infertility is diagnosed. However, literature is currently inconsistent in its recommendations for patients with myomas who are seeking fertility treatment. The Practice Committee of the American Society for Reproductive Medicine (ASRM) created a guideline paper that thoroughly discusses the research centered around fertility and leiomyomas.[24] The authors are verbose in their censure of the literature and the difficulty in drawing clear conclusions about true links between subfertility and uterine leiomyomas. Criticisms include variations in types of fibroids studied, ages of patients seeking pregnancy, and inconsistency in whether the patients are undergoing assisted reproductive technology (ART) or attempting spontaneous pregnancy. Also, some studies include submucosal fibroids and others do not. Some articles look only at patients with intramural or subserosal fibroids. Without consistency in the type of fibroids studied, it is difficult to understand what role the type of fibroid plays in infertility. Cassini and colleagues reported fertility improvement from 27% to 43% after hysteroscopic resection of type 0 fibroids.[86][87] Size is another confounder in appropriately studying fibroids; patients can have one large, solitary fibroid or multiple, small fibroids both of which can distort reproductive anatomy in their own way. In a study of 168 women with at least one fibroid greater than 5 cm in size, without distortion of the endometrial cavity, removal still offered positive impacts on ART.[88] In an RCT of patients with at least one intramural fibroid $\leq$4 cm in size, removal did not improve fertility outcomes.[86] Fortunately with all this debate, there are studies that show the removal of subserosal and intramural fibroids does not have a negative impact on fertility.[89] A recent study echoed this finding but with submucosal leiomyomas stating that patients who have undergone surgical correction have similar pregnancy outcomes overall to those patients who have not undergone surgery.[90] Practitioners should be aware of the lack of data to support a correlation between fibroids and subfertility. We seek to better understand the type, size, and symptoms that indicate the need for myomectomy in the patient undergoing workup for subfertility.

## SUMMARY

Submucosal fibroids have been implicated in AUB and can be associated with subfertility. Accurate characterization of the fibroids with imaging studies and hysteroscopy is essential to guide the management strategies. Hysteroscopic myomectomy is a safe and effective minimally invasive option for submucosal myomas, with excellent results. Several technological advances have recently been introduced to improve the safety and efficiency of the procedure, even as an office hysteroscopic procedure in the proper setting and with adequate training.

## CLINICS CARE POINTS

- Hysteroscopic myomectomy should be used for removal of all intrauterine fibroids including types 2 and 3 fibroids
- Appropriate workup for patients includes history, physical examination, imaging, and shared decision-making concerning patient's desire for future fertility or uterine-sparing surgery
- Practitioners should be familiar with the available technology for hysteroscopic myomectomy and their various indications (ie, cold loop dissection, resectoscopic surgery, and tissue removal systems)
- Optimizing safety and visualization during a procedure is critical, it is important to prepare especially for cases of large submucosal leiomyomas
- Clinicians performing hysteroscopic myomectomy should be able to quickly diagnose and correct common, sometimes morbid, complications of this procedure
- If safety is compromised or if no further intervention can be performed, a multistep procedure is appropriate
- There is a lack of consensus about fibroids and infertility; hysteroscopic myomectomy does appear to improve pregnancy outcomes but does not have the same positive impact on reducing miscarriage rates

## DISCLOSURE

N.S. Moawad: Consultant, Cooper Surgical, Inc, and Myovant Sciences; H. Palin: Nothing to disclose.

## SUPPLEMENTARY DATA

Supplementary data related to this article can be found online at https://doi.org/10.1016/j.ogc.2022.02.012.

## REFERENCES

1. van Dongen H, de Kroon CD, Jacobi CE, et al. Diagnostic hysteroscopy in abnormal uterine bleeding: a systematic review and meta-analysis. BJOG 2007;114(6):664–75 [published Online First: Epub Date]].
2. Kim JJ, Sefton EC. The role of progesterone signaling in the pathogenesis of uterine leiomyoma. Mol Cell Endocrinol 2012;358(2):223–31 [published Online First: Epub Date]].

3. Reis FM, Bloise E, Ortiga-Carvalho TM. Hormones and pathogenesis of uterine fibroids. Best Pract Res Clin Obstet Gynaecol 2016;34:13–24 [published Online First: Epub Date]|.

4. Bulun SE, Simpson ER, Word RA. Expression of the CYP19 gene and its product aromatase cytochrome P450 in human uterine leiomyoma tissues and cells in culture. J Clin Endocrinol Metab 1994;78(3):736–43. https://doi.org/10.1210/jcem.78.3.8126151 [published Online First: Epub Date]|.

5. Shao R, Fang L, Xing R, et al. Differential expression of estrogen receptor alpha and beta isoforms in multiple and solitary leiomyomas. Biochem Biophys Res Commun 2015;468(1–2):136–42 [published Online First: Epub Date]|.

6. Bakas P, Liapis A, Vlahopoulos S, et al. Estrogen receptor alpha and beta in uterine fibroids: a basis for altered estrogen responsiveness. Fertil Steril 2008;90(5):1878–85 [published Online First: Epub Date]|.

7. Bulun SE, Moravek MB, Yin P, et al. Uterine leiomyoma stem cells: linking progesterone to growth. Semin Reprod Med 2015;33(5):357–65 [published Online First: Epub Date]|.

8. Ishikawa H, Ishi K, Serna VA, et al. Progesterone is essential for maintenance and growth of uterine leiomyoma. Endocrinology 2010;151(6):2433–42 [published Online First: Epub Date]|.

9. Peddada SD, Laughlin SK, Miner K, et al. Growth of uterine leiomyomata among premenopausal black and white women. Proc Natl Acad Sci U S A 2008;105(50):19887–92 [published Online First: Epub Date]|.

10. Cramer SF, Patel A. The frequency of uterine leiomyomas. Am J Clin Pathol 1990;94(4):435–8 [published Online First: Epub Date]|.

11. Ishikawa H, Reierstad S, Demura M, et al. High aromatase expression in uterine leiomyoma tissues of African-American women. J Clin Endocrinol Metab 2009;94(5):1752–6 [published Online First: Epub Date]|.

12. Chiaffarino F, Parazzini F, La Vecchia C, et al. Diet and uterine myomas. Obstet Gynecol 1999;94(3):395–8 [published Online First: Epub Date]|.

13. Tinelli A, Vinciguerra M, Malvasi A, et al. Uterine Fibroids and Diet. Int J Environ Res Public Health 2021;18(3) [published Online First: Epub Date]|.

14. He Y, Zeng Q, Dong S, et al. Associations between uterine fibroids and lifestyles including diet, physical activity and stress: a case-control study in China. Asia Pac J Clin Nutr 2013;22(1):109–17 [published Online First: Epub Date]|.

15. Stewart EA, Cookson CL, Gandolfo RA, et al. Epidemiology of uterine fibroids: a systematic review. BJOG 2017;124(10):1501–12 [published Online First: Epub Date]|.

16. Eggert SL, Huyck KL, Somasundaram P, et al. Genome-wide linkage and association analyses implicate FASN in predisposition to Uterine Leiomyomata. Am J Hum Genet 2012;91(4):621–8 [published Online First: Epub Date]|.

17. Wallach EE, Vlahos NF. Uterine myomas: an overview of development, clinical features, and management. Obstet Gynecol 2004;104(2):393–406 [published Online First: Epub Date]|.

18. Nishino M, Togashi K, Nakai A, et al. Uterine contractions evaluated on cine MR imaging in patients with uterine leiomyomas. Eur J Radiol 2005;53(1):142–6 [published Online First: Epub Date]|.

19. Stewart EA, Nowak RA. Leiomyoma-related bleeding: a classic hypothesis updated for the molecular era. Hum Reprod Update 1996;2(4):295–306 [published Online First: Epub Date]|.

20. Piecak K, Milart P. Hysteroscopic myomectomy. Prz Menopauzalny 2017;16(4):126–8 [published Online First: Epub Date]|.

21. Donnez J, Jadoul P. What are the implications of myomas on fertility? a need for a debate? Hum Reprod 2002;17(6):1424–30 [published Online First: Epub Date]|.
22. Somigliana E, Reschini M, Bonanni V, et al. Fibroids and natural fertility: a systematic review and meta-analysis. Reprod Biomed Online 2021;43(1):100–10 [published Online First: Epub Date]|.
23. Chaker A, Ferchiou M, Lahmar MM, et al. [Uterine fibromyomas: fertility after myomectomy. About 41 cases]. Tunis Med 2004;82(12):1075–81.
24. Practice Committee of the American Society for Reproductive Medicine. Electronic address Aao, practice committee of the american society for reproductive m. removal of myomas in asymptomatic patients to improve fertility and/or reduce miscarriage rate: a guideline. Fertil Steril 2017;108(3):416–25 [published Online First: Epub Date]|.
25. Davis BJ, Haneke KE, Miner K, et al. The fibroid growth study: determinants of therapeutic intervention. J Womens Health (Larchmt) 2009;18(5):725–32 [published Online First: Epub Date]|.
26. Laughlin-Tommaso SK, Hesley GK, Hopkins MR, et al. Clinical limitations of the International federation of gynecology and obstetrics (FIGO) classification of uterine fibroids. Int J Gynaecol Obstet 2017;139(2):143–8 [published Online First: Epub Date]|.
27. Munro MG, Critchley HO, Broder MS, et al. FIGO classification system (PALM-COEIN) for causes of abnormal uterine bleeding in nongravid women of reproductive age. Int J Gynaecol Obstet 2011;113(1):3–13 [published Online First: Epub Date]|.
28. Lasmar RB, Lasmar BP, Celeste RK, et al. A new system to classify submucous myomas: a Brazilian multicenter study. J Minim Invasive Gynecol 2012;19(5): 575–80 [published Online First: Epub Date]|.
29. Lasmar RB, Xinmei Z, Indman PD, et al. Feasibility of a new system of classification of submucous myomas: a multicenter study. Fertil Steril 2011;95(6):2073–7 [published Online First: Epub Date]|.
30. Dueholm M, Lundorf E, Hansen ES, et al. Accuracy of magnetic resonance imaging and transvaginal ultrasonography in the diagnosis, mapping, and measurement of uterine myomas. Am J Obstet Gynecol 2002;186(3):409–15 [published Online First: Epub Date]|.
31. Sabry ASA, Fadl SA, Szmigielski W, et al. Diagnostic value of three-dimensional saline infusion sonohysterography in the evaluation of the uterus and uterine cavity lesions. Pol J Radiol 2018;83:e482–90 [published Online First: Epub Date]|.
32. Salim R, Lee C, Davies A, et al. A comparative study of three-dimensional saline infusion sonohysterography and diagnostic hysteroscopy for the classification of submucous fibroids. Hum Reprod 2005;20(1):253–7 [published Online First: Epub Date]|.
33. Levens ED, Wesley R, Premkumar A, et al. Magnetic resonance imaging and transvaginal ultrasound for determining fibroid burden: implications for research and clinical care. Am J Obstet Gynecol 2009;200(5):537 e1–7 [published Online First: Epub Date]|.
34. Sakala MD, Carlos RC, Mendiratta-Lala M, et al. Understanding patient preference in female pelvic imaging: transvaginal ultrasound and MRI. Acad Radiol 2018;25(4):439–44 [published Online First: Epub Date]|.
35. Kresowik JD, Syrop CH, Van Voorhis BJ, et al. Ultrasound is the optimal choice for guidance in difficult hysteroscopy. Ultrasound Obstet Gynecol 2012;39(6):715–8 [published Online First: Epub Date]|.

36. Laughlin-Tommaso SK, Lu D, Thomas L, et al. Short-term quality of life after myomectomy for uterine fibroids from the COMPARE-UF fibroid registry. Am J Obstet Gynecol 2020;222(4):345 e1–45, e22 [published Online First: Epub Date]|.

37. Berger U, Altgassen C, Kuss S, et al. Patients' satisfaction with laparoscopic myomectomy. J Psychosom Obstet Gynaecol 2006;27(4):225–30 [published Online First: Epub Date]|.

38. Hart R, Molnar BG, Magos A. Long term follow up of hysteroscopic myomectomy assessed by survival analysis. Br J Obstet Gynaecol 1999;106(7):700–5 [published Online First: Epub Date]|.

39. Bettocchi S, Di Spiezio Sardo A, Ceci O, et al. A new hysteroscopic technique for the preparation of partially intramural myomas in office setting (OPPIuM technique): a pilot study. J Minim Invasive Gynecol 2009;16(6):748–54 [published Online First: Epub Date]|.

40. Cancado RD, Munoz M. Intravenous iron therapy: how far have we come? Rev Bras Hematol Hemoter 2011;33(6):461–9 [published Online First: Epub Date]|.

41. Macdougall IC. Evolution of iv iron compounds over the last century. J Ren Care 2009;35(Suppl 2):8–13 [published Online First: Epub Date]|.

42. Celik H, Sapmaz E. Use of a single preoperative dose of misoprostol is efficacious for patients who undergo abdominal myomectomy. Fertil Steril 2003;79(5):1207–10 [published Online First: Epub Date]|.

43. Iavazzo C, Mamais I, Gkegkes ID. Use of misoprostol in myomectomy: a systematic review and meta-analysis. Arch Gynecol Obstet 2015;292(6):1185–91 [published Online First: Epub Date]|.

44. Pakrashi T. New hysteroscopic techniques for submucosal uterine fibroids. Curr Opin Obstet Gynecol 2014;26(4):308–13 [published Online First: Epub Date]|.

45. Ferrero S, Scala C, Vellone VG, et al. Preoperative treatment with ulipristal acetate before outpatient hysteroscopic myomectomy. Gynecol Obstet Invest 2020;85(2):178–83 [published Online First: Epub Date]|.

46. Vitale SG, Ferrero S, Caruso S, et al. Ulipristal Acetate Before Hysteroscopic Myomectomy: A Systematic Review. Obstet Gynecol Surv 2020;75(2):127–35 [published Online First: Epub Date]|.

47. Lethaby A, Puscasiu L, Vollenhoven B. Preoperative medical therapy before surgery for uterine fibroids. Cochrane Database Syst Rev 2017;11:CD000547 [published Online First: Epub Date]|.

48. Parazzini F, Vercellini P, De Giorgi O, et al. Efficacy of preoperative medical treatment in facilitating hysteroscopic endometrial resection, myomectomy and metroplasty: literature review. Hum Reprod 1998;13(9):2592–7 [published Online First: Epub Date]|.

49. Favilli A, Mazzon I, Grasso M, et al. Intraoperative effect of preoperative gonadotropin-releasing hormone analogue administration in women undergoing cold loop hysteroscopic myomectomy: a randomized controlled trial. J Minim Invasive Gynecol 2018;25(4):706–14 [published Online First: Epub Date]|.

50. Muzii L, Boni T, Bellati F, et al. GnRH analogue treatment before hysteroscopic resection of submucous myomas: a prospective, randomized, multicenter study. Fertil Steril 2010;94(4):1496–9 [published Online First: Epub Date]|.

51. Mencaglia L, Tantini C. GnRH agonist analogs and hysteroscopic resection of myomas. Int J Gynaecol Obstet 1993;43(3):285–8 [published Online First: Epub Date]|.

52. Soon R, Tschann M, Salcedo J, et al. Paracervical block for laminaria insertion before second-trimester abortion: a randomized controlled trial. Obstet Gynecol 2017;130(2):387–92 [published Online First: Epub Date]|.

53. Asgari Z, Razavi M, Hosseini R, et al. Evaluation of paracervical block and iv sedation for pain management during hysteroscopic polypectomy: a randomized clinical trial. Pain Res Manag 2017;2017:5309408 [published Online First: Epub Date]|.

54. Tangsiriwatthana T, Sangkomkamhang US, Lumbiganon P, et al. Paracervical local anaesthesia for cervical dilatation and uterine intervention. Cochrane Database Syst Rev 2013;9:CD005056 [published Online First: Epub Date]|.

55. Sahay N, Agarwal M, Bara M, et al. Deep sedation or paracervical block for daycare gynecological procedures: a prospective, comparative study. Gynecol Minim Invasive Ther 2019;8(4):160–4 [published Online First: Epub Date]|.

56. Wong ASW, Cheung CW, Yeung SW, et al. Transcervical intralesional vasopressin injection compared with placebo in hysteroscopic myomectomy: a randomized controlled trial. Obstet Gynecol 2014;124(5):897–903 [published Online First: Epub Date]|.

57. Frishman G. Vasopressin: if some is good, is more better? Obstet Gynecol 2009; 113(2 Pt 2):476–7 [published Online First: Epub Date]|.

58. Morrison DM. Management of hysteroscopic surgery complications. AORN J 1999;69(1):194–7, 99-197; quiz 10, 13-197, 21.

59. Stamatellos I, Koutsougeras G, Karamanidis D, et al. Results after hysteroscopic management of premenopausal patients with dysfunctional uterine bleeding or intrauterine lesions. Clin Exp Obstet Gynecol 2007;34(1):35–8.

60. Berg A, Sandvik L, Langebrekke A, et al. A randomized trial comparing monopolar electrodes using glycine 1.5% with two different types of bipolar electrodes (TCRis, Versapoint) using saline, in hysteroscopic surgery. Fertil Steril 2009;91(4): 1273–8 [published Online First: Epub Date]|.

61. Mencaglia L, Lugo E, Consigli S, et al. Bipolar resectoscope: the future perspective of hysteroscopic surgery. Gynecol Surg 2008;6(1):15 [published Online First: Epub Date]|.

62. Mazzon I, Favilli A, Grasso M, et al. Is cold loop hysteroscopic myomectomy a safe and effective technique for the treatment of submucous myomas with intramural development? a series of 1434 surgical procedures. J Minim Invasive Gynecol 2015;22(5):792–8 [published Online First: Epub Date]|.

63. Di Spiezio Sardo A, Calagna G, Di Carlo C, et al. Cold loops applied to bipolar resectoscope: A safe "one-step" myomectomy for treatment of submucosal myomas with intramural development. J Obstet Gynaecol Res 2015;41(12): 1935–41 [published Online First: Epub Date]|.

64. van Wessel S, van Vliet H, Schoot BC, et al. Hysteroscopic morcellation versus bipolar resection for removal of type 0 and 1 submucous myomas: a randomized trial. Eur J Obstet Gynecol Reprod Biol 2021;259:32–7 [published Online First: Epub Date]|.

65. Yin X, Cheng J, Ansari SH, et al. Hysteroscopic tissue removal systems for the treatment of intrauterine pathology: a systematic review and meta-analysis. Facts Views Vis Obgyn 2018;10(4):207–13.

66. Vitale SG, Sapia F, Rapisarda AMC, et al. Hysteroscopic morcellation of submucous myomas: a systematic review. Biomed Res Int 2017;2017:6848250 [published Online First: Epub Date]|.

67. Mazzon I, Favilli A, Grasso M, et al. Predicting success of single step hysteroscopic myomectomy: a single centre large cohort study of single myomas. Int J Surg 2015;22:10–4 [published Online First: Epub Date]|.

68. Arnold A, Ketheeswaran A, Bhatti M, et al. A prospective analysis of hysteroscopic morcellation in the management of intrauterine pathologies. J Minim Invasive Gynecol 2016;23(3):435–41 [published Online First: Epub Date]|.
69. Litta P, Leggieri C, Conte L, et al. Monopolar versus bipolar device: safety, feasibility, limits and perioperative complications in performing hysteroscopic myomectomy. Clin Exp Obstet Gynecol 2014;41(3):335–8.
70. Friedman JA, Wong JMK, Chaudhari A, et al. Hysteroscopic myomectomy: a comparison of techniques and review of current evidence in the management of abnormal uterine bleeding. Curr Opin Obstet Gynecol 2018;30(4):243–51 [published Online First: Epub Date]|.
71. Liang Y, Ren Y, Wan Z, et al. Clinical evaluation of improved MyoSure hysteroscopic tissue removal system for the resection of type II submucosal myomas. Medicine (Baltimore) 2017;96(50):e9363 [published Online First: Epub Date]|.
72. Shazly SA, Laughlin-Tommaso SK, Breitkopf DM, et al. Hysteroscopic morcellation versus resection for the treatment of uterine cavitary lesions: a systematic review and meta-analysis. J Minim Invasive Gynecol 2016;23(6):867–77 [published Online First: Epub Date]|.
73. Meulenbroeks D, Hamerlynck TW, Saglam-Kara S, et al. Hysteroscopic tissue removal systems: a randomized in vitro comparison. J Minim Invasive Gynecol 2017;24(1):159–64 [published Online First: Epub Date]|.
74. Umranikar S, Clark TJ, Saridogan E, et al. BSGE/ESGE guideline on management of fluid distension media in operative hysteroscopy. Gynecol Surg 2016;13(4):289–303 [published Online First: Epub Date]|.
75. Worldwide AAMIG, Munro MG, Storz K, et al. AAGL practice report: practice guidelines for the management of hysteroscopic distending media: (replaces hysteroscopic fluid monitoring guidelines. J Am Assoc Gynecol Laparosc. 2000;7:167-168.). J Minim Invasive Gynecol 2013;20(2):137–48 [published Online First: Epub Date]|.
76. Istre O, Bjoennes J, Naess R, et al. Postoperative cerebral oedema after transcervical endometrial resection and uterine irrigation with 1.5% glycine. Lancet 1994;344(8931):1187–9 [published Online First: Epub Date]|.
77. Sterns RH. Disorders of plasma sodium–causes, consequences, and correction. N Engl J Med 2015;372(1):55–65 [published Online First: Epub Date]|.
78. Stoloff DR, Isenberg RA, Brill AI. Venous air and gas emboli in operative hysteroscopy. J Am Assoc Gynecol Laparosc 2001;8(2):181–92 [published Online First: Epub Date]|.
79. Dyrbye BA, Overdijk LE, van Kesteren PJ, et al. Gas embolism during hysteroscopic surgery using bipolar or monopolar diathermia: a randomized controlled trial. Am J Obstet Gynecol 2012;207(4):271 e1–6 [published Online First: Epub Date]|.
80. Capmas P, Levaillant JM, Fernandez H. Surgical techniques and outcome in the management of submucous fibroids. Curr Opin Obstet Gynecol 2013;25(4):332–8 [published Online First: Epub Date]|.
81. Lasmar RB, Barrozo PR, Dias R, et al. Submucous myomas: a new presurgical classification to evaluate the viability of hysteroscopic surgical treatment–preliminary report. J Minim Invasive Gynecol 2005;12(4):308–11 [published Online First: Epub Date]|.
82. Loddo A, Djokovic D, Drizi A, et al. Hysteroscopic myomectomy: the guidelines of the international society for gynecologic endoscopy (ISGE). Eur J Obstet Gynecol Reprod Biol 2022;268:121–8 [published Online First: Epub Date]|.

83. Zayed M, Fouda UM, Zayed SM, et al. Hysteroscopic myomectomy of large sub-mucous myomas in a 1-step procedure using multiple slicing sessions technique. J Minim Invasive Gynecol 2015;22(7):1196–202 [published Online First: Epub Date]|.

84. Korkmazer E, Tekin B, Solak N. Ultrasound guidance during hysteroscopic myo-mectomy in G1 and G2 Submucous Myomas: for a safer one step surgery. Eur J Obstet Gynecol Reprod Biol 2016;203:108–11 [published Online First: Epub Date]|.

85. Ludwin A, Ludwin I, Pitynski K, et al. Transrectal ultrasound-guided hysteroscopic myomectomy of submucosal myomas with a varying degree of myometrial pene-tration. J Minim Invasive Gynecol 2013;20(5):672–85 [published Online First: Epub Date]|.

86. Casini ML, Rossi F, Agostini R, et al. Effects of the position of fibroids on fertility. Gynecol Endocrinol 2006;22(2):106–9 [published Online First: Epub Date]|.

87. Pritts EA, Parker WH, Olive DL. Fibroids and infertility: an updated systematic re-view of the evidence. Fertil Steril 2009;91(4):1215–23 [published Online First: Epub Date]|.

88. Bulletti C, Dez D, Levi Setti P, et al. Myomas, pregnancy outcome, and in vitro fertilization. Ann N Y Acad Sci 2004;1034:84–92 [published Online First: Epub Date]|.

89. Guillaume J, Benjamin F, Jean-Gilles M, et al. Myomectomy and tuboplasty per-formed at the same time in cases of distal tubal obstruction with associated fi-broids. J Reprod Med 2000;45(6):461–4.

90. Fonge YN, Carter AS, Hoffman MK, et al. Obstetrical outcomes are unchanged after hysteroscopic myomectomy in women with submucosal fibroids. Am J Ob-stet Gynecol MFM 2020;2(4):100192 [published Online First: Epub Date]|.

# Evaluation and Management of Common Intraoperative and Postoperative Complications in Gynecologic Endoscopy

Brittany Lees, MD*, Jubilee Brown, MD

## KEYWORDS

- Complications • Injury • Laparoscopy

## KEY POINTS

- Safe trocar placement is essential to avoid injury, and immediate recognition of trocar injury is essential.
- Urologic injury can involve the bladder or ureters and must be recognized and repaired immediately to avoid more complex repairs or urinoma or fistula formation.
- Bowel injury may be subtle, and delayed presentation is common. Vigilance in the postoperative setting is necessary to diagnose injury and allow timely repair.

## INTRODUCTION

Laparoscopy was first pioneered by Jacobaeus in the early 1900s, and it has evolved to include a variety of specialized platforms and techniques, including conventional laparoscopy, single-incision laparoscopy, and robotics.[1] A recent review article reported complication rates using a variety of definitions and concluded that adverse events are reported to occur between 0.2% and 18% of conventional gynecologic laparoscopy and 3% and 15% of robot-assisted gynecologic procedures. Although major complication rates were similar between laparotomy and laparoscopy, there was a lower incidence of minor complications at 15.2% versus 4.3% to 8.9%, respectively.[2] The relatively low complication rates make some details difficult to study. This article seeks to highlight the most current complication rates, outline steps toward prevention of complications, and detail management of key complications related to minimally invasive surgery (MIS) in gynecology.

Division of Gynecologic Oncology, Levine Cancer Institute at Atrium Health, 1021 Morehead Medical Drive, Suite 2100, Charlotte, NC 28204, USA
* Corresponding author.
*E-mail address:* brittany.lees@atriumhealth.org

Obstet Gynecol Clin N Am 49 (2022) 355–368
https://doi.org/10.1016/j.ogc.2022.03.002
0889-8545/22/© 2022 Elsevier Inc. All rights reserved.

obgyn.theclinics.com

## LAPAROSCOPIC ENTRY

A majority of laparoscopic complications occur at the time of intraabdominal entry. Complications include injury to structures, such as the bowel, bladder, or liver; preperitoneal insufflation; failure to achieve pneumoperitoneum; and puncture of the pregnant uterus.[3–6] The risk of vascular injury at the time of entry is approximately 3 per 1000 surgical case.[7] Bowel injury incidence ranges between 0.13% and 0.54%, with 37.3% to 55% occurring during entry. Although 75% of injuries are to the small bowel, colonic injury or gastric perforation also can occur.[8]

Techniques for abdominal entry include Veress needle placement, direct optical entry, and the open or Hasson technique. Each of these entry techniques can be utilized in the umbilical, supraumbilical, or left-upper quadrant (Palmer point) areas, and the location typically is chosen based on avoiding areas of prior surgery or avoiding the area of a large adnexal or uterine mass. Each technique and location have individual pros and cons that require careful review of patient anatomy and prior surgical history.

The Veress needle has an external diameter of 2 mm and, therefore, is smaller compared with 5 mm to 12 mm for other trocars. Thus, any resultant injury is smaller than with other entry techniques.[9] Direct visualization and open (or Hasson) entry techniques have overall low rates of reported complications and theoretically seem safer by avoiding blind entry. Despite the purported advantages of individual techniques, a 2019 Cochrane Review reported insufficient evidence to demonstrate differences in the rates of failed entry, vascular injury, visceral injury, or other major complications between open-entry and closed-entry techniques.[10] There also was insufficient evidence to demonstrate differences in the rates of vascular or visceral injury between direct vision entry and Veress needle entry. The reviewers noted moderate evidence for a reduction in risk of failed entry with direct trocar insertion compared with Veress needle access, but the data were not limited to gynecologic cases, and many of the studies included in the review excluded patients with a high body mass index (BMI) and previous abdominal surgery[9] (**Table 1**).

### Abdominal Wall Injuries

Abdominal wall injuries at the time of trocar insertion include vascular injury to the inferior epigastric artery and neuropathy secondary to injury to the iliohypogastric and ilioinguinal nerves. A thorough understanding of anatomy is important to avoid either complication.

Injury to the inferior epigastric artery has an incidence of approximately 3 per 1000 surgical cases.[7] Prevention of injury involves vascular identification and avoiding trocar placement along its expected route. Cadaveric studies have demonstrated many potential origins of the inferior epigastric artery; it typically arises from the external iliac artery but also can arise from the femoral or obturator artery.[11] The first key step to avoiding injury is identification of the inferior epigastric vessels through direct laparoscopic inspection of the anterior abdominal wall after initial port placement, but this may not be possible in the setting of high BMI.[7,12] In general, placement of lateral trocars greater than 7 cm from the midline helps to avoid injury. Care should be taken to not track medially on the fascia at the time of entry (see **Table 1**). Techniques to manage incidental inferior epigastric arterial injury include direct bipolar coagulation or sealing of the vessel, tension with a balloon trocar, placement of a foley catheter balloon with pressure to tamponade, cut-down below the rectus muscle to achieve direct ligation of the vessel superior and inferior to the injury, and laparoscopic suture ligation of the vessel superior and inferior to the injury, either with a laparoscopic straight ligature carrier, laparoscopic ligation, or temporary mattress suture placement[13] (**Table 2**).

| Table 1 Techniques to avoid complications | |
|---|---|
| **Category of Injury** | **Strategy to Avoid Injury** |
| Trocar insertion | Direct entry has decrease in failure rate compared with Veress entry<br>No other comparative advantage for any specific technique |
| Inferior epigastric vessels | Transillumination<br>Direct inspection<br>Placement of trocar >7 cm lateral to midline |
| Ilioinguinal or iliohypogastric nerve | Placement of lateral trocars ≥2 cm above and medial to ASIS |
| Vascular injury (aorta/vena cava) | Initial trocar insertion at an angle appropriate for the patient's BMI<br>Initial trocar insertion with the operating table flat |
| Bowel injury | Insert trocars at a relaxed, level position<br>Thorough understanding of anatomy and surgical history<br>Review prior operative reports prior to deciding on entry site<br>Consider access in right upper quadrant with orogastric tube in place for any patient with prior midline or periumbilical surgery |
| Trocar site hernia | Close fascia at any port site ≥10 mm |
| Bladder injury | Backfill bladder when necessary to define location<br>Lateral approach to dissection when significant scarring |
| Ureteral injury | Careful anatomic dissection and identification<br>Cephalad displacement of the uterine manipulator<br>Maintain surgical dissection fundal to the manipulator ring<br>Consider stents or lighted stents in select cases |
| Neurologic injury | Careful positioning, padding, avoid extreme extension/flexion<br>Clear identification of obturator nerve in obturator space |
| VCD | Laparoscopic closure has lower risk than vaginal closure<br>Minimize cautery artifact<br>Sutures should be ≥5 mm deep and ≤5 mm apart |
| Port site metastasis | Avoid repeated removal and replacement of trocars<br>Use containment systems for cancer-containing specimens |

Rates of injury to the ilioinguinal and iliohypogastric nerves are not well documented, and overall neurologic injury is cited at less than 2%, but one study showed injury to these nerves as high as 4.9% when fascial closure is required in lateral port sites.[14,15] Preventing injury is challenging because the nerves cannot be visualized directly, so knowledge of anatomy is essential to prevent injury to these nerves. A study of cadavers identified the ilioinguinal nerve to be located an average of 3.1 cm medial and 3.7 cm inferior to the anterior superior iliac spine (ASIS). The iliohypogastric nerve was located within 2.1 cm medial and 0.9 cm inferior to the ASIS.[16] Therefore, placement of the lateral tracers at least 2 cm above and medial to the ASIS should avoid incidental nerve injury (see **Table 1**). Injury to these nerves typically

| Table 2 | |
|---|---|
| **Management of laparoscopic complications** | |
| **Category of Injury** | **Management Strategy** |
| Inferior epigastric vessels | Direct bipolar coagulation or sealing of the vessel<br>Tamponade with a balloon trocar or Foley catheter<br>Laparoscopic suture placement proximal and distal to the injury<br>Direct ligation with cut-down |
| Ilioinguinal or iliohypogastric nerve | Supportive care<br>Release of surrounding sutures<br>Trigger point injections |
| Vascular injury (aorta/vena cava) | Emergent laparotomy (in most cases) |
| Bowel injury | Immediate repair with possible resection and reanastomosis<br>Observation in some cases of injury <2 mm with a Veress needle |
| Trocar site hernia | Reduce hernia and surgically repair fascia |
| Bladder injury | Double-layer watertight closure with absorbable suture<br>Postoperative Foley catheter placement<br>No antibiotics indicated |
| Ureteral injury | Dependent on type and location of injury |
| Neurologic injury | Supportive care, physical therapy, analgesics<br>Direct repair for transections (eg, obturator nerve) |
| VCD | Immediate repair, typically through vaginal approach<br>Consider laparoscopic or abdominal evaluation in select cases |

manifests as a burning or sharp pain in the location of the port site that is not responsive to narcotic therapy. Management depends on the degree of discomfort and suspected cause of injury. Typically, medical management with neuropathic pain medications or lidocaine, and time improves symptoms. If no improvement and a fascial stitch is suspected as the source, however, surgical intervention for stitch removal should be considered[15] (see **Table 2**).

## Vascular Injuries

Deeper vessels also can be injured with laparoscopic entry but are rare, with a rate of 0.2/1000 procedures.[17] Any periumbilical entry technique requires consideration of the varying anatomic layout of the bifurcation of the aorta and vena cava, depending on body habitus. The bifurcation of the aorta in thin patients often is just deep to the umbilicus, whereas in obese patients the bifurcation often is cephalad to the umbilicus.[18] Therefore, the operating table should be flat (no Trendelenburg), and insertion of the Veress needle or optical trocar must be at a 30° angle in patients with a normal BMI and must be vertical in obese patients to avoid injury to the great vessels (see **Table 1**). If the great vessels are pierced with either the Veress needle or a trocar, emergent laparotomy is indicated for immediate repair, because this situation can be catastrophic (see **Table 2**). It is imperative to alert the anesthesia team and operating room staff, obtain blood products, begin fluid resuscitation, hold compression to minimize further volume depletion, and engage in primary repair or consult vascular surgery, depending on the surgeon's skills.

Mesenteric or omental vascular injury also can occur at time of trocar placement. Such injuries can be prevented through meticulous technique with appropriate pressure upon entry, avoiding areas of prior surgical incisions, and using an upper abdominal entry site. Management may include observation once additional ports are placed, coagulation with a sealing device, or suture ligation of the injured vessel, but care should be taken to avoid bowel injury during repair. Hemostasis must be confirmed under low or no pressure before the case is completed.[17]

## Bowel Injuries

The incidence of bowel injury is 0.13% to 0.54%, and one-third to one-half of these injuries occur at the time of laparoscopic entry. Although 75% of injuries are to the small bowel, colonic injury or gastric perforation also can occur. The mortality rate from gastrointestinal injury is as high as 3.6%.[19] Regardless of entry technique, having the patient in the appropriate relaxed, level position and a thorough understanding of anatomy and surgical history should be considered prior to proceeding with entry. Consideration should be given to access in the right upper quadrant for any patient with prior midline or periumbilical surgery. Previous operative reports should be reviewed prior to a decision on initial port site placement (see **Table 1**).

The most important part of minimizing morbidity and mortality from bowel injury is intraoperative recognition. Unfortunately, 41% of bowel injuries are identified in a delayed manner.[19] In order to help ensure recognition, the camera should look directly at the bowel in the vector of entry to ensure no injury, and, prior to exiting the case, the camera should be inserted through a secondary port and the site of entry should be inspected. If an injury is identified or the entry is difficulty, the surgeon should ensure there has not been a through and through perforation across both sides of the bowel lumen. Injury from Veress insertion may be indicated by foul smelling gas through the needle, reflux of bowel contents through the Veress needle, high insufflation pressures, or asymmetrical abdominal distension.[20] A small 2 mm Veress perforation may not require repair.[21,22] Trocar injuries which are larger in caliber, have irregular borders, or are leaking bowel contents require immediate repair or resection with reanastamosis (see **Table 2**). The decision to proceed with laparoscopic versus open repair is dependent on surgeon preference and expertise. Specific surgical repair techniques are beyond the scope of this review.

An additional trocar-related gastrointestinal injury is postoperative port site hernia formation, which has an incidence of 0.17% to 1.5%.[23,24] Hernias rarely occur in ports that are smaller than 10 mm and usually are limited to port sites with a diameter of at least 10 mm. Therefore, prevention of port site hernias requires fascial closure of any port site greater than or equal to 10 mm at the completion of the case.[25-28] Although recommended, such fascial closure does not negate the possibility of port site herniation.[24] Single-incision laparoscopic techniques, also employed in gynecologic surgery, require a larger midline incision and have a higher rate of incisional hernia.[29] The use of bladeless trocars also protects against hernia formation, as a systematic review demonstrated lower rates of port site herniation with bladeless trocars24 (see **Table 1**). Diagnosis of a port site hernia is suggested by pain at the site, nausea or vomiting, tenderness, and a bulge on physical examination. Presentation can mirror that of a partial small bowel obstruction or ileus. Computerized tomography (CT) scan findings can confirm clinical suspicion. Management requires surgical reduction of the hernia and fascial repair; bowel resection is limited to cases in which the bowel has been strangulated or devascularized with compromised viability.[30] Incarcerated hernias require emergent surgery (see **Table 2**).

## GASTROINTESTINAL INJURIES

The incidence of bowel injury during MIS is 0.13% to 0.54%,[19] with most injuries occurring to the small bowel. In addition to injury during abdominal entry or trocar placement, bowel injuries can occur during dissection. Risk factors include the presence of adhesions, prior surgeries with resultant distorted anatomy, and tumor or endometriotic implants involving the bowel.

The key to prevention is the use of meticulous sharp dissection without cautery when operating near the small or large bowel. Thermal injury can occur even without adhesive disease or direct dissection due to lateral thermal spread of energy devices or incidental contact with a hot instrument.

It is imperative to have a high level of suspicion for bowel injury, particularly when significant enterolysis is performed. An intraoperative bubble test can be performed to exclude either small or large bowel injury. To evaluate the rectosigmoid, saline is instilled into the pelvis, and the large bowel is occluded gently with pressure cephalad to the area of presumed injury; air is instilled into the rectum with a proctoscope or bulb suction; and the pool of saline is inspected for air bubbles as the colon expands with insufflation. A lack of bubbles is reassuring but does not guarantee the lack of a thermal injury or deserosalization. To evaluate the small bowel, saline is instilled into the abdomen or pelvis; the area of bowel with the suspected injury is submerged in the saline pool with bowel graspers. Small bowel contents are pushed across the area and the pool of saline is inspected for air bubbles or succus.

Bowel injuries less than 1 cm typically can be repaired with interrupted, delayed, absorbable sutures placed perpendicular to the axis of the bowel to avoid stricture. Full-thickness injuries require a double-layer closure. Larger injuries and most thermal injuries require resection with reanastamosis. Repair can be performed laparoscopically or the patient can be converted to a small mini-laparotomy or a larger laparotomy depending on the surgeon's expertise, location of the injury, and mobility of the affected area of the bowel.[31]

Bowel injury potentially can be catastrophic when not recognized intraoperatively.[31] Postoperatively, patients present with nausea, vomiting, pain, fever, abdominal pain or distention, and/or leukocytosis. It is imperative that any concerning symptoms be investigated with CT of the abdomen and pelvis with oral and IV contrast. If a perforation is identified, immediate surgical exploration usually is indicated with a washout and repair of the affected area. Colostomy or protective ileostomy may be indicated, depending on the type and location of injury[31] (see **Table 2**).

## UROLOGIC INJURIES

The anatomic locations of the ureter and bladder in the pelvis lead to a higher risk of injury in gynecologic surgery compared with other types of surgery. The risk of urinary tract injury is estimated at 0.33% for all benign gynecologic conditions and up to 1% with laparoscopic hysterectomy.[32–34] Bladder injuries are slightly more common than ureteral injuries, with a rate estimated at 0.24% (range, 0.05%–1.8%) for all benign gynecologic conditions and 0.66% with laparoscopic hysterectomy (range, 0.05%–1.8%).[21,22] Ureteral injuries are estimated to occur in 0.02% to 1.5% of laparoscopic gynecologic procedures.[22,32,35–37]

### Bladder Injury

Because the urinary bladder sits anterior to the uterus and cervix, injuries typically occur following extensive lysis of adhesions, such as in women with multiple prior cesarean or other pelvic surgeries.[38] Risk factors also include endometriosis, urinary tract anomalies, prior pelvic irradiation, uterine size over 250 g, and obesity. Certain indications for surgery also increase the risk of injury, including prolapse, urinary incontinence, leiomyomata, or a large pelvic mass.[35,38] It is controversial whether cancer surgery is an independent risk factor for urologic injury.[35]

Cystotomies typically are recognized intraoperatively and occur most often at the dome of the bladder. Strategies for prevention focus on intraoperative identification of the bladder. This can be performed by filling the bladder with saline or carbon dioxide in order to distend it and better identify its borders. In the setting of significant fibrosis, a lateral approach to dissection can help identify a clear plane for dissection that is not embedded in scar tissue (see **Table 1**). Bladder injury can be obvious when there is large cystotomy with visualization of Foley balloon. Occult bladder injury can present with hematuria, distended Foley bag, or extravasation of urine in the surgical field.[39] Concern for bladder injury should be investigated intraoperatively by backfilling the bladder through the Foley catheter with 300 mL of methylene blue or indigo carmine diluted with saline. Sterile milk also may be used. Cystoscopy may help identify a smaller perforation, bleeding, or suture within the bladder.[39]

When injuries involve the dome of the bladder, the size of the defect dictates management. Defects less than 2 mm can be managed expectantly. Defects between 2 mm and 10 mm can be managed with repair or with catheter drainage for 5 days to 7 days. Defects over 1 cm require repair. Repair typically can be performed laparoscopically by experienced surgeons, as long as there is adequate visualization and there is no involvement of the trigone or bladder neck. Repair is performed with 2 layers of absorbable suture (3-0 then 2-0 Vicryl or Monocryl) placed full thickness to incorporate the bladder mucosa. This double-layer closure incorporates the mucosa in the first layer and an imbricating suture of the muscularis over the second layer. Sutures can be either interrupted or running, and barbed suture also is acceptable. The repair should be watertight and tested for integrity with retrograde fill of the bladder prior to completion of the laparoscopic portion of the procedure. A Foley catheter should remain postoperatively for 5 days to 14 days, depending on the size and location of the injury, because re-epithelialization occurs in 3 days to 4 days and normal strength is regained by 21 days[40] (see **Table 2**). Limited data support the use of postoperative antibiotic use.[41,42] Prior to catheter removal, a CT cystogram and a voiding trial may be performed.

### Ureteral Injury

Ureteral injuries, although less common than bladder injuries, are diagnosed more frequently postoperatively and often are the result of thermal injury or suture entrapment.[33] The three most common locations of ureteral injury are the pelvic brim during transection of the infundibulopelvic ligament and ligation of the gonadal (ovarian) vessels, the cardinal ligament near the uterine vessels during dissection or coagulation of the uterine vessels, and the ureterovesical junction during bladder dissection or vaginal cuff closure. Ureters also can be devascularized during extensive ureterolysis.

Transperitoneal visualization and/or retroperitoneal dissection and identification of the ureter throughout its course during surgery are the keys to prevention of ureteral injury during gynecologic surgery. When ligating the gonadal vessels, often a retroperitoneal approach with a window made between the gonadal vessels, and the ureter allows the surgeon to cauterize the vessels with adequate space from the ureter to avoid injury. Although the ureter is typically approximately 2 cm anterolateral to the cervix, it can be as close as 0.5 cm in some women.[43] Vermiculation must be visualized to ensure that the ureter is identified accurately. The surgeon must take care to stay above the level of the cervicovaginal junction, a location that corresponds to the delineation of the Koh ring or cup, and the assistant should continually exert cephalad pressure on the uterine manipulator to maximize the distance from the cervix to the ureter. The surgeon should be aware of thermal spread associated with sealing devices, which range from 0 mm to 22 mm, depending on the device, activation time, and settings.[44] The bladder also should be adequately dissected away from the upper vagina to allow appropriate closure without injury. Placement of preoperative ureteral stents may be useful to identify the ureters in selected cases, but data do not show a consistent advantage to this strategy[45–47] (see **Table 1**).

Identification of many ureteral injuries can be accomplished by intravenous (IV) instillation of indigo carmine or preoperative oral phenazopyridine.[39] If colored fluid is seen to pool in the pelvis, a bladder or ureteral transection is noted and the location must be identified in order to effect repair. Thermal and devascularization injuries can be more challenging to identify intraoperatively. Recent data support the use of near infrared imaging with indocyanine green to identify devascularization injuries.[48] Cystoscopy also may be performed at the completion of the procedure in order to identify brisk bilateral ureteral jets; a single dose of preoperative oral Pyridium (100–200 mg), 1 mL of diluted IV sodium fluorescein (1 mL of 10% fluorescein diluted in 9 mL saline), IV indigo carmine, or IV or intravesical methylene blue may be utilized, but this not always is necessary because the urine jets may be visualized without any additional dye. If bilateral jets are not identified initially, additional time may be allocated, the patient may be given additional fluid or furosemide or placed into reverse Trendelenburg position or a temporary ureteral stent may be placed to ensure patency.[39] If an injury is still suspected, an intraoperative IV pyelogram or retrograde cystogram may be performed.[39] Early detection decreases the risk of requiring reimplantation by tenfold.[49]

The type of injury—kinking, ligation, crush, or thermal—and the location of the injury determine the necessary repair strategy. Crush injuries, delayed thermal injuries, and partial obstructions can be difficult to recognize.[43] If the ureter is kinked by a suture, the ureter can be dissected away, or the surgeon can remove the offending suture, assess ureteral integrity, and place a stent if any abnormality in appearance or efflux is noted.[50] If the ureter has been clamped, the surgeon should immediately remove the clamp and inspect the ureter for integrity. Next, a ureteral stent should be placed for 2 weeks to 6 weeks, and given the potential for urine leakage with extensive injury, a drain should be placed to prevent urinoma for at least 7 days to 10 days.[49] For both thermal injuries and crush injuries, if the ureter is viable, then a ureteral stent may be placed, and no further repair is required. If the ureter is not viable, then resection of the necrotic segment is indicated with reattachment either to the ureter or reimplantation in the bladder is indicated (discussed later). Thermal injuries may have associated cellular damage past the visible area of injury, and this may lead to delayed disruption if not recognized intraoperatively. The location of the injury also determines the strategy for repair. In general, an injury below the pelvic brim that requires resection of a segment of the ureter requires reimplantation into the bladder, usually with a lengthening technique, such as the psoas hitch or a Boari flap. Injuries above the pelvic brim may require direct ureteroureterostomy or transureteroureterostomy[50,51] (see **Table 2**). Although the general gynecologist may repair bladder injuries, it is within the scope of practice of a subspecialist or urologist to repair most ureteral injuries.

Delayed diagnosis of a ureteral or bladder injury may present with flank pain, costovertebral tenderness, unexplained fever, persistent ileus, a lower abdominal mass (urinoma), urine leakage from the vagina, decreased urine output, or unexplained hematuria.[52] These findings should prompt cystoscopy, a CT cystogram, renal ultrasound, retrograde pyelogram, and/or CT of the abdomen and pelvis. Once a ureteral obstruction is identified, retrograde stent placement should be attempted, and, if unable to be passed, antegrade stents may be attempted, although percutaneous nephrostomy tubes may be required. Any infection should be treated, and catheterization of the urinary bladder may be required to stop urine leakage.

The routine use of cystoscopy following laparoscopic hysterectomy has been debated in the gynecologic literature and unfortunately no prospective randomized data exist to determine benefit. Most surgeons would agree that although cystoscopy does not eliminate the potential for a postoperatively identified injury, in complicated dissections or with any suspicion of injury, cystoscopy should be considered and is cost-effective.[53–55]

## NEUROLOGIC INJURIES

Neurologic injuries are estimated to occur in less than 2% of gynecologic procedures and are not unique to the laparoscopic approach.[56,57] A vast majority are related to improper positioning and prolonged surgical time and include both upper and lower extremity neuropathies. The most common nerve injuries are the peroneal, femoral, lateral femoral cutaneous, obturator, and ulnar nerves.[14] Prevention includes appropriate positioning and padding to avoid stretch and compression.

Upper extremity nerve injury typically is due to excessive stretch of the brachial plexus from improper positioning, with an incidence of 0.16%.[58] It is vital to ensure that patients' arms are placed in a neutral position at their sides with adequate padding along the ulnar nerve with relaxed hand positioning. Some surgeons, particularly with obese patients, use shoulder straps to minimize cephalad displacement when in steep Trendelenburg. Caution should be used because these can place lateral pressure on the brachial plexus and prevent proper movement of the shoulders should the patient slide cephalad. A crossed-strap approach is recommended to minimize this risk[59] (see **Table 1**). Brachial plexus injuries can present with both motor and sensory deficits, depending on the nerve root distribution injured. Early physical therapy and neurology consultation is recommended, especially when motor deficits occur. Oral analgesics, epileptics, and vitamin B can be prescribed for sensory discomforts[60] (see **Table 2**).

Lower extremity injuries from positioning include the femoral, lateral femoral cutaneous, obturator, and sciatic nerves. In general, injury occurs from prolonged dorsal lithotomy position with hip flexion, abduction, or external rotation. Prior to draping, the surgeon should ensure that patients' (1) hips are flexed between 60° and 170°; (2) knees are flexed between 90° and 120°; (3) hips are abducted no more than 90°; and (4) hips are minimally externally rotated.[56] Prolonged operative time has been shown to increase the risk of nerve injury.[61] With cases longer than 2 hours, the surgeon should pause periodically to ensure that appropriate positioning has been maintained. Management of compression or stretch injuries typically involves observation with supportive care, neurology consultation, and physical therapy.

Aside from direct nerve injury at the time of trocar placement or fascial suturing, direct nerve injury or severing of the genitofemoral, obturator, or sciatic nerves can occur with retroperitoneal dissection. Due to their anatomic locations, these nerves are more likely to be injured with retroperitoneal dissections for advanced pathology associated with endometriosis, leiomyoma, and pelvic masses as well as with lymphadenectomies and pelvic floor repairs.[57] During dissection of the obturator space, the obturator nerve always should be identified clearly (see **Table 1**). When transections are identified at the time of surgery, immediate repair should be undertaken. The nerve ends can be reapproximated with 5-0 Prolene to encourage regrowth; this may require the assistance of a neurosurgeon to ensure proper alignment of the nerve.[62] When noted after surgery and felt to be a crush or compression injury, typically supportive care with early physical therapy and pain control is warranted. Physical therapy is necessary for most patients, and most patients regain function. Most injuries have complete recovery, particularly with early recognition (see **Table 2**).

## VAGINAL CUFF DEHISCENCE

Hysterectomy is the most frequently performed major gynecologic surgery and has the unique complication of vaginal cuff dehiscence (VCD). The incidence of VCD is relatively low and occurs in 0.14% to 4.1% of cases, which has made it difficult to study.[63] Laparoscopic procedures have slightly higher rates of VCD compared with laparotomy or vaginal hysterectomy,[64] but robotic and laparoscopic platforms appear similar.[65,66] The type of closure, including suture type, single-layered versus double-layered closure, or vaginal versus laparoscopic approach, all have been examined, and most data are retrospective. A 2015 systematic review and meta-analysis showed no difference between barbed and conventional suture.[67] More recent studies have demonstrated no difference in cuff complications, including dehiscence, related to suture type, including nonabsorbable suture.[68,69] A recent randomized control trial of 1408 patients demonstrated an increased rate of dehiscence with transvaginal as opposed to laparoscopic closure (1% vs 2.7%; odds ratio 2.78; 95%, CI 1.16–6.62; $P = .01$).[70] A 2021 meta-analysis concluded that a laparoscopic approach with barbed suture yielded the least risk for VCD.[66] In terms of best practice for cuff closure to minimize VCD, there exists no randomized controlled trial, although many experts believe minimizing cautery effect and taking sufficient bites at least 5 mm deep and no more than 5 mm apart with peritoneal closure could minimize complications[71] (see **Table 1**). Risk factors from trials do note an increase in dehiscence among premenopausal women and smokers.[70]

Patients with VCD can present at any time after surgery, with studies showing variability from 2 weeks to more than 5 years.[63] Presenting signs and symptoms can include pelvic or abdominal pain, vaginal bleeding or discharge, vaginal mass, or pressure. The surgical urgency and route of repair depends on the size of the defect, clinical status of the patient, extent of bleeding, and bowel involvement. VCD repair typically is performed through a vaginal or laparoscopic approach but also can be done abdominally. No data suggest the superiority of any specific route or repair method. Surgeons should ensure that additional associated problems, including bowel ischemia or intraabdominal abscess, are assessed adequately. The vaginal tissue edges should be trimmed to ensure healthy tissue that is reapproximated with good strength.[63] Infections should be treated, and patients should be counseled regarding any modifiable risk factors and extended pelvic rest (see **Table 2**).

## SUMMARY

MIS, through conventional multiport, single-port, or robotic platforms, will continue to become more prevalent in gynecologic surgery, given the significant improvements in perioperative outcomes. It is important for surgeons to be cognizant of potential complications when undertaking any of these techniques. Although a vast majority of surgical complications occur on entry, no specific entry technique currently is recommended over another. Surgeons should be aware of strategies for prevention, diagnosis, and treatment of bowel, vascular, neurologic, and urinary tract injuries.

## DISCLOSURE

Dr B. Lees has no commercial or financial conflicts of interest and there are no funding sources. Dr J. Brown has participated in the Speakers' Bureau for Clovis and for Eisai and has received funding for this. Dr J. Brown has participated in advisory boards or as a consultant with Caris, Biodesix, Janssen, Tempus, Olympus, Clovis, Invitae, and GSK/Tesaro. Dr J. Brown has participated in research with GSK/Tesaro and Genentech.

## REFERENCES

1. Sutton C, Abbott J. History of power sources in endoscopic surgery. J Minim Invasive Gynecol 2013;20(3):271–8.
2. Watrowski R, Kostov S, Alkatout I. Complications in laparoscopic and robotic-assisted surgery: definitions, classifications, incidence and risk factors - an up-to-date review. Wideochir Inne Tech Maloinwazyjne 2021;16(3):501–25.
3. Jansen FW, Kapiteyn K, Trimbos-Kemper T, et al. Complications of laparoscopy: a prospective multicentre observational study. Br J Obstet Gynaecol 1997;104(5):595–600.
4. Jansen FW, Kolkman W, Bakkum EA, et al. Complications of laparoscopy: an inquiry about closed- versus open-entry technique. Am J Obstet Gynecol 2004;190(3):634–8.
5. Segura-Sampedro JJ, Cañete-Gómez J, Reguera-Rosal J, et al. Unnoticed biloma due to liver puncture after Veress needle insertion. Ann Med Surg (Lond) 2015;4(3):238–9.
6. Post RJ, Friedrich E, Amaya KE, et al. Inadvertent Perforation of a Gravid Uterus During Laparoscopy. JSLS 2019;23(3).
7. Lavery S, Porter S, Trew G, et al. Use of inferior epigastric artery embolization to arrest bleeding at operative laparoscopy. Fertil Steril 2006;86(3):719.e13-4.
8. Sharp Howard T. Diagnostic and Operative Laparoscopy. In: Jones Howard W, Rock John A, editors. Te Linde's operative gynecology. Philadelphia: Wolters Kluwer; 2015. p. 281–3.
9. Vilos GA, Ternamian A, Dempster J, et al. No. 193-Laparoscopic Entry: A Review of Techniques, Technologies, and Complications. J Obstet Gynaecol Can 2017;39(7):e69–84.
10. Ahmad G, Duffy JM, Phillips K, et al. Laparoscopic entry techniques. Cochrane Database Syst Rev 2019;1:CD006583.
11. Rao MP, Swamy V, Arole V, et al. Study of the course of inferior epigastric artery with reference to laparoscopic portal. J Minim Access Surg 2013;9(4):154–8.
12. Quint EH, Wang FL, Hurd WW. Laparoscopic transillumination for the location of anterior abdominal wall blood vessels. J Laparoendosc Surg 1996;6(3):167–9.
13. de Rosnay P, Chandiramani S, Owen E. Injury of epigastric vessels at laparoscopy: diagnosis and management. Gynecol Surg 2011;8(3):353–6.
14. Abdalmageed OS, Bedaiwy MA, Falcone T. Nerve Injuries in Gynecologic Laparoscopy. J Minim Invasive Gynecol 2017;24(1):16–27.
15. Shin JH, Howard FM. Abdominal wall nerve injury during laparoscopic gynecologic surgery: incidence, risk factors, and treatment outcomes. J Minim Invasive Gynecol 2012;19(4):448–53.
16. Whiteside JL, Barber MD, Walters MD, et al. Anatomy of ilioinguinal and iliohypogastric nerves in relation to trocar placement and low transverse incisions. Am J Obstet Gynecol 2003;189(6):1574–8 [discussion: 1578].

17. Asfour V, Smythe E, Attia R. Vascular injury at laparoscopy: a guide to management. J Obstet Gynaecol 2018;38(5):598–606.

18. Hurd WW, Bude RO, DeLancey JO, et al. The relationship of the umbilicus to the aortic bifurcation: implications for laparoscopic technique. Obstet Gynecol 1992; 80(1):48–51.

19. Llarena NC, Shah AB, Milad MP. Bowel injury in gynecologic laparoscopy: a systematic review. Obstet Gynecol 2015;125(6):1407–17.

20. Berry MA, Rangraj M. Conservative treatment of recognized laparoscopic colonic injury. JSLS 1998;2(2):195–6.

21. Almeida OD Jr, Val-Gallas JM. Small trocar perforation of the small bowel: a case report. JSLS 1998;2(3):289–90.

22. Reich H. Laparoscopic bowel injury. Surg Laparosc Endosc 1992;2(1):74–8.

23. Kadar N, Reich H, Liu CY, et al. Incisional hernias after major laparoscopic gynecologic procedures. Am J Obstet Gynecol 1993;168(5):1493–5.

24. Gutierrez M, Stuparich M, Behbehani S, et al. Does closure of fascia, type, and location of trocar influence occurrence of port site hernias? A literature review. Surg Endosc 2020;34(12):5250–8.

25. Lambertz A, Stüben BO, Bock B, et al. Port-site incisional hernia - A case series of 54 patients. Ann Med Surg (Lond) 2017;14:8–11.

26. Boone JD, Fauci JM, Barr ES, et al. Incidence of port site hernias and/or dehiscence in robotic-assisted procedures in gynecologic oncology patients. Gynecol Oncol 2013;131(1):123–6.

27. Diez-Barroso R Jr, Palacio CH, Martinez JA, et al. Robotic port-site hernias after general surgical procedures. J Surg Res 2018;230:7–12.

28. Seamon LG, Backes F, Resnick K, et al. Robotic trocar site small bowel evisceration after gynecologic cancer surgery. Obstet Gynecol 2008;112(2 Pt 2):462–4.

29. Hoyuela C, Juvany M, Guillaumes S, et al. Long-term incisional hernia rate after single-incision laparoscopic cholecystectomy is significantly higher than that after standard three-port laparoscopy: a cohort study. Hernia 2019;23(6):1205–13.

30. Kwon YH, Choe EK, Ryoo SB, et al. Long-Term Surgical Outcome of Trocar Site Hernia Repair. Am Surg 2017;83(2):176–82.

31. Eisner IS, Wadhwa RK, Downing KT, et al. Prevention and management of bowel injury during gynecologic laparoscopy: an update. Curr Opin Obstet Gynecol 2019;31(4):245–50.

32. Adelman MR, Bardsley TR, Sharp HT. Urinary tract injuries in laparoscopic hysterectomy: a systematic review. J Minim Invasive Gynecol 2014;21(4):558–66.

33. Wong JMK, Bortoletto P, Tolentino J, et al. Urinary Tract Injury in Gynecologic Laparoscopy for Benign Indication: A Systematic Review. Obstet Gynecol 2018; 131(1):100–8.

34. Unger CA, Walters MD, Ridgeway B, et al. Incidence of adverse events after uterosacral colpopexy for uterovaginal and posthysterectomy vault prolapse. Am J Obstet Gynecol 2015;212(5):603–7.

35. Teeluckdharry B, Gilmour D, Flowerdew G. Urinary Tract Injury at Benign Gynecologic Surgery and the Role of Cystoscopy: A Systematic Review and Meta-analysis. Obstet Gynecol 2015;126(6):1161–9.

36. Brummer TH, Seppala TT, Harkki PS. National learning curve for laparoscopic hysterectomy and trends in hysterectomy in Finland 2000-2005. Hum Reprod 2008;23(4):840–5.

37. Makinen J, Brummer T, Jalkanen J, et al. Ten years of progress–improved hysterectomy outcomes in Finland 1996-2006: a longitudinal observation study. BMJ Open 2013;3(10):e003169.

38. Wallis CJ, Cheung DC, Garbens A, et al. Occurrence of and Risk Factors for Uro-logical Intervention During Benign Hysterectomy: Analysis of the National Surgi-cal Quality Improvement Program Database. Urology 2016;97:66–72.

39. Hurt WJI, CM. Intraoperative ureteral injuries and urinary diversion. In: Nichols D, editor. Gynecologic and Obstetric surgery. Baltimore: Mosby; 1993. p. 900–10.

40. Yeomans ER, Hoffman Larry C, Gilstrap GF III. Cunnigham and Gilstrap's Oper-ative Obstetrics. 3rd edition. McGraw Hill; 1995.

41. ACOG practice bulletin No. ACOG practice bulletin No. 104: antibiotic prophy-laxis for gynecologic procedures. Obstet Gynecol 2009;113(5):1180–9.

42. Lusardi G, Lipp A, Shaw C. Antibiotic prophylaxis for short-term catheter bladder drainage in adults. Cochrane Database Syst Rev 2013;(7):CD005428.

43. Hurd WW, Chee SS, Gallagher KL, et al. Location of the ureters in relation to the uterine cervix by computed tomography. Am J Obstet Gynecol 2001;184(3): 336–9.

44. Einarsson, J.G., J, Overview of Electrosurgery, in UpToDate, K. Collins, Editor. 2011: Waltham, MA.

45. Merritt AJ, Crosbie EJ, Charova J, et al. Prophylactic pre-operative bilateral ureteric catheters for major gynaecological surgery. Arch Gynecol Obstet 2013; 288(5):1061–6.

46. Schimpf MO, Gottenger EE, Wagner JR. Universal ureteral stent placement at hysterectomy to identify ureteral injury: a decision analysis. BJOG 2008;115(9): 1151–8.

47. Wood EC, Maher P, Pelosi MA. Routine use of ureteric catheters at laparoscopic hysterectomy may cause unnecessary complications. J Am Assoc Gynecol Lap-arosc 1996;3(3):393–7.

48. Raimondo D, Borghese G, Mabrouk M, et al. Use of Indocyanine Green for Intra-operative Perfusion Assessment in Women with Ureteral Endometriosis: A Prelim-inary Study. J Minim Invasive Gynecol 2021;28(1):42–9.

49. Wu HH, Yang PY, Yeh GP, et al. The detection of ureteral injuries after hysterec-tomy. J Minim Invasive Gynecol 2006;13(5):403–8.

50. Stanhope CR, Wilson TO, Utz WJ, et al. Suture entrapment and secondary ure-teral obstruction. Am J Obstet Gynecol 1991;164(6 Pt 1):1513–9 [discussion: 1517–9].

51. Wright JE, Handa VL. Operative Injuries to the Ureter, in Te Linde's operative gy-necology, H.I.R, III. Philadelphia: Jones; 2015. p. 932–43.

52. Sakellariou P, Protopapas AG, Voulgaris Z, et al. Management of ureteric injuries during gynecological operations: 10 years experience. Eur J Obstet Gynecol Re-prod Biol 2002;101(2):179–84.

53. Cadish LA, Ridgeway BM, Shepherd JP. Cystoscopy at the time of benign hyster-ectomy: a decision analysis. Am J Obstet Gynecol 2019;220(4):369.e7.

54. Vakili B, Chesson RR, Kyle BL, et al. The incidence of urinary tract injury during hysterectomy: a prospective analysis based on universal cystoscopy. Am J Ob-stet Gynecol 2005;192(5):1599–604.

55. Worldwide, A.A.M.I.G., AAGL Practice Report: Practice guidelines for intraoper-ative cystoscopy in laparoscopic hysterectomy. J Minim Invasive Gynecol 2012;19(4):407–11.

56. Barnett JC, Hurd WW, Rogers RM, et al. Laparoscopic positioning and nerve in-juries. J Minim Invasive Gynecol 2007;14(5):664–73 [quiz: 673].

57. Cardosi RJ, Cox CS, Hoffman MS. Postoperative neuropathies after major pelvic surgery. Obstet Gynecol 2002;100(2):240–4.

58. Romanowski L, Reich H, McGlynn F, et al. Brachial plexus neuropathies after advanced laparoscopic surgery. Fertil Steril 1993;60(4):729–32.
59. Shveiky D, Aseff JN, Iglesia CB. Brachial plexus injury after laparoscopic and robotic surgery. J Minim Invasive Gynecol 2010;17(4):414–20.
60. Finnerup NB, Attal N, Haroutounian S, et al. Pharmacotherapy for neuropathic pain in adults: a systematic review and meta-analysis. Lancet Neurol 2015; 14(2):162–73.
61. Warner MA, Martin JT, Schroeder DR, et al. Lower-extremity motor neuropathy associated with surgery performed on patients in a lithotomy position. Anesthesiology 1994;81(1):6–12.
62. Vasilev SA. Obturator nerve injury: a review of management options. Gynecol Oncol 1994;53(2):152–5.
63. Cronin B, Sung VW, Matteson KA. Vaginal cuff dehiscence: risk factors and management. Am J Obstet Gynecol 2012;206(4):284–8.
64. Hur HC, Donnellan N, Mansuria S, et al. Vaginal cuff dehiscence after different modes of hysterectomy. Obstet Gynecol 2011;118(4):794–801.
65. Dauterive E, Morris G. Incidence and characteristics of vaginal cuff dehiscence in robotic-assisted and traditional total laparoscopic hysterectomy. J Robot Surg 2012;6(2):149–54.
66. Uccella S, Zorzato PC, Kho RM. Incidence and Prevention of Vaginal Cuff Dehiscence after Laparoscopic and Robotic Hysterectomy: A Systematic Review and Meta-analysis. J Minim Invasive Gynecol 2021;28(3):710–20.
67. Bogliolo S, Musacchi V, Dominoni M, et al. Barbed suture in minimally invasive hysterectomy: a systematic review and meta-analysis. Arch Gynecol Obstet 2015;292(3):489–97.
68. Lopez CC, Ríos JFL, González Y, et al. Barbed suture versus conventional suture for vaginal cuff closure in total laparoscopic hysterectomy: randomized controlled clinical trial. J Minim Invasive Gynecol 2019;26(6):1104–9.
69. MacKoul P, Danilyants N, Sarfoh V, et al. A Retrospective Review of Vaginal Cuff Dehiscence: Comparing Absorbable and Nonabsorbable Sutures. J Minim Invasive Gynecol 2020;27(1):122–8.
70. Uccella S, Malzoni M, Cromi A, et al. Laparoscopic vs transvaginal cuff closure after total laparoscopic hysterectomy: a randomized trial by the Italian Society of Gynecologic Endoscopy. Am J Obstet Gynecol 2018;218(5):500.e13.
71. O'Hanlan KA, Emeney PL, Peters A, et al. Analysis of a Standardized Technique for Laparoscopic Cuff Closure following 1924 Total Laparoscopic Hysterectomies. Minim Invasive Surg 2016;2016:1372685.

# Abdominal Wall Endometriosis

Christine E. Foley, MD[a,*], Patricia Giglio Ayers, MD[a], Ted T. Lee, MD[b]

## KEYWORDS

- Abdominal wall endometriosis • Rectus muscle endometriosis
- Incisional endometriosis

## KEY POINTS

- Prior abdominal surgery, specifically history of cesarean delivery, is the largest risk factor for abdominal wall endometriosis (AWE).
- Cyclic abdominal pain, a palpable mass, and history of abdominal surgery is the pathognomonic triad for the clinical presentation of AWE.
- Abdominal ultrasonography is the first-line imaging modality for AWE; however, MRI should be considered for nodules greater than 3 cm to guide surgical management.
- Surgical approach depends on lesion size and location, with an abdominal approach preferred for superficial disease and a laparoscopic approach preferred when the bulk of disease is subfascial or involving the rectus muscle.
- Following surgical excision, patients' symptoms improve with a low recurrence rate.

## INTRODUCTION

Endometriosis, defined as the presence of endometrial glands and stroma outside the uterine cavity, occurs in up to 10% of reproductive age women.[1] The pathogenesis of endometriosis is likely multifactorial, including factors such as ectopic endometrial tissue, altered immunity, imbalanced cell proliferation and apoptosis, aberrant endocrine signaling, and genetics.[2] Abdominal wall endometriosis (AWE) is a specific type of extrapelvic endometriosis in which the glands and stroma of the endometrium are found within the layers of the abdominal wall. The incidence is reported to be 0.3% to 3.5%.[3–7] It is hypothesized that endometrial cells are transported and deposited into the abdominal incision via surgical instrumentation and proliferate within the abdominal wall.[8] However, this hypothesis does not account for all cases of AWE,

[a] Department of Obstetrics and Gynecology, Warren Alpert Medical School of Brown University, Women & Infants Hospital, 101 Dudley Street, Providence, RI 02905, USA; [b] Department of Obstetrics, Gynecology, and Reproductive Sciences, University of Pittsburgh School of Medicine, UPMC Magee-Womens Hospital, 300 Halket Street, Pittsburgh, PA 15213, USA
* Corresponding author.
E-mail address: Christine.e.foley@gmail.com
Twitter: docfoleygyn (C.E.F.); tedleefly (T.T.L.)

Obstet Gynecol Clin N Am 49 (2022) 369–380
https://doi.org/10.1016/j.ogc.2022.02.013
obgyn.theclinics.com

because sporadic cases in patients with no prior surgical history are reported in the literature.[9–11] Alternative hypotheses of lymphatic or hematogenous dissemination may account for cases with no surgical history.[4]

## CLINICAL PRESENTATION

Similar to pelvic endometriosis, the diagnosis of AWE requires a high level of clinical suspicion. Patients are of reproductive age and present with a single mass.[12] The mean time from initial surgery to symptomatic AWE ranges from months to years.[4,5,12] Cyclic abdominal pain, a palpable mass, and a history of abdominal surgery is the pathognomonic triad, but individual cases may vary in presentation.[13] Up to 90% of patients will report cyclic abdominal pain as their primary symptom.[4,12,14] Cyclic symptoms are caused by fluctuations in the menstrual cycle with hormonal stimulation driving cell proliferation, swelling, and bleeding.[15] Patients also experience noncyclic pain and focal pain with palpation of a mass. Not all cases present with a palpable nodule, and the physical examination can be limited by body habitus. New research suggests that body mass index is an additional risk factor for AWE, making the clinical diagnosis of AWE all the more challenging.[4,16]

Focal abdominal wall tenderness close to a prior incision should increase the clinical suspicion for AWE because 80% to 90% of cases are associated with a surgical scar.[4] More than 80% of patients with AWE have a history of a cesarean delivery, and the apices of cesarean incisions are the most common location for implants. The implant can appear distant from the Pfannenstiel skin incision secondary to the lateral and superior extension of the fascia relative to the skin during cesarean delivery.[17] AWE located in surgical scars is reported after other pelvic surgeries such as abdominal myomectomies, hysterectomies, laparoscopic pelvic surgery, appendectomies, and hernia repairs.[4,18] Not all AWE cases have a history of prior surgery.[9–11,19,20] Common sites of spontaneous AWE include the groin/inguinal (58%), umbilicus (36%), and less commonly the rectus muscle (3%).[21,22] AWE that occurs in the absence of prior abdominal surgery is associated with pelvic endometriosis.[4] A thorough history followed by a complete abdominal, pelvic, and rectal examination is necessary to determine the extent of pelvic endometriosis in cases of sporadic AWE.

Lack of a palpable abdominal mass on examination does not exclude AWE and could suggest subfascial disease involving the rectus muscle. Rectus muscle endometriosis (RME) is a specific subtype of AWE in which ectopic endometrial tissue is located within the body of the rectus muscle.[20] RME can be isolated to the rectus muscle or can be an extension of AWE involving the subcutaneous tissue and fascia. In a single-institution case series of RME, Melnyk and colleagues[19] reported that whereas 91% had focal abdominal tenderness on examination, only 54% had palpable nodules, reflecting the subfascial location of the disease. Patients also reported pain with movements that strain the rectus muscle such as coughing, sneezing, or performing a sit-up, which can help differentiate subfascial from superficial disease.[19]

## DIAGNOSIS

The differential diagnosis of AWE includes incisional hernias, lipomas, abscesses, granulomas, cysts, sarcoma, and scar tissue.[5,13,23] AWE should be included in the differential diagnosis of women with a symptomatic mass even without a history of biopsy-proven endometriosis. Final diagnosis is made after pathologic examination, but imaging is useful to narrow the differential.

## Imaging

Imaging eliminates other causes of an abdominal wall mass and provides the clinician with information on the size, depth, and extent of fascial involvement to guide surgical planning.[14] First-line imaging is abdominal wall ultrasonography because this is a low-cost, readily available imaging modality. Abdominal ultrasonography can also exclude abdominal wall hernias.[23] On ultrasonography, AWE appears cystic, solid, or mixed (**Fig. 1**) and power Doppler demonstrates internal vascularity.[6,8,23] In a series of 151 cases of AWE, Zhang and Liu[18] reported a preoperative detection rate of 97% with abdominal ultrasound. Abdominal ultrasonography can distinguish subcutaneous and subfascial disease, with a reported 92% sensitivity identifying endometriosis involving the rectus body.[6] Zhang and colleagues reported a lower rate of accuracy for depth of invasion at 26.5% and described lower accuracy for size of the lesion.[18] Therefore, for AWE lesions 3 cm or larger or nodules that are difficult to palpate, the authors recommend MRI to define the location and depth of the endometriosis nodule, providing a map for surgical intervention. The authors also recommend MRI if the patient has no history of abdominal surgery, because these patients have increased rates of concurrent deep infiltrating endometriosis of the pelvis.

On MRI, AWE implants are solid hypointense or slightly hyperintense on T2- and T1 fat-suppressed images with small areas of hemorrhage appearing hyperintense compared with the surrounding abdominal wall (**Fig. 2**).[24] Recent hemorrhage displays as high signal intensity on T1- and T2-weighted images, and hemosiderin deposits show low signal intensity on T1- and T2-weighted images.[8] Various protocols for AWE are reported in the literature without consensus for the role of diffusion-weighted images and intravenous (IV) contrast.[24] Computed tomography (CT) has less clinical benefit. On CT with IV contrast, AWE typically enhances; however, the exact characteristics depend on the menstrual cycle phase, proportion of stromal and glandular tissue, and extent of surrounding inflammation and fibrosis.[8] CT findings are generally nonspecific, and we do not recommend their routine clinical use for the workup of suspected AWE.

Ultrasound-guided fine-needle aspiration (FNA) can be used to confirm suspected AWE as an alternate to surgical removal. FNA is a minimally invasive, rapid procedure that can exclude malignancy before planned surgical intervention.[6] Abdominal wall hernia must be ruled out with ultrasonography before performing FNA. Histologic confirmation can be inconclusive due to fibrosis and limited tissue available for sampling.[6,25,26] In one large study, 75% of cases were inconclusive.[25] We recommend

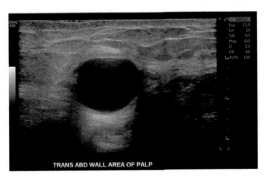

**Fig. 1.** Transabdominal ultrasonography with hypoechoic nodule in the cesarean delivery scar. Final pathology demonstrated abdominal wall endometriosis (AWE).

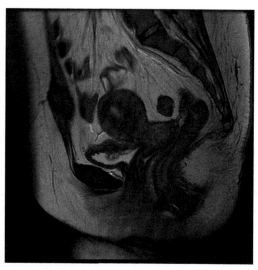

**Fig. 2.** AWE in the cesarean delivery scar on MRI.

FNA as an additional diagnostic tool when a patient's history and imaging is not conclusive or concerning for malignancy.

## MANAGEMENT
### Expectant

Patients who are asymptomatic or whose AWE is an incidental finding may be managed expectantly. We do not recommend routine imaging surveillance for asymptomatic individuals. Additional workup or treatment can be initiated in response to new symptoms.[27]

### Medical

Medical management can be offered to patients as a conservative approach. Continuous combined oral contraceptive pills (OCPs), progestins, or Gonadotropin-releasing hormone agonists suppress ovulation and produce a hypoestrogenic state; this can relieve symptoms but does not decrease the size of lesions.[3] The overall success of medical management is temporary, with symptom recurrence following drug discontinuation. Medications can be used temporarily as a bridge to surgery or menopause to optimize symptom relief.

### Ablation

Recent small, retrospective studies demonstrate the safety and feasibility of high-intensity focused ultrasound (HIFU) ablation for AWE.[28] Ultrasound-guided HIFU ablates AWE through coagulative tissue necrosis caused by ultrasound pressure-induced heat in the focused area.[28] The 6- and 12-month outcomes show decreased lesion size and lower pain scores with no differences in pain-free relief between patients treated with HIFU compared with those treated with surgical excision.[29,30] Advantages of HIFU include shorter hospital stays, no structural disruption to the abdominal wall layers, and minimal blood loss.[30] Thermal ablation with CT- or ultrasound-guided cryoablative needles is also described in the literature.[31,32] Long-term symptomatic relief from this procedure remains unknown with only 1 nonrandomized study comparing outcomes with surgical excision.[31] Both techniques are promising for the nonsurgical management of AWE; however, large prospective comparative studies are necessary.[3]

## Surgical

Surgical excision remains the standard of care for the treatment of symptomatic AWE. Endometriosis nodules are removed via wide local excision and an abdominal incision. Experts recommend surgical margins of at least 1 cm to ensure complete disease resection.[7,17] During surgery, the endometriosis is easily delineated from the surrounding abdominal wall based off texture and appearance. The firm, fibrotic tissue is typically pink and can have cystic areas of blue, purple, or brown (**Fig. 3**). About 60% to 70% of reported cases involve the fascia, which requires repair after excision.[4,12,14] As described later, primary fascial repair is performed for small defects (<3 cm). Experts recommend fascial repair with mesh for lesions greater than 3 cm.[3,17] Preoperative imaging is crucial to determine the size and location of the endometriosis, allowing for a planned multidisciplinary approach with general or plastic surgery for large nodules involving the fascia. If RME is less than 2 cm and without obvious physical landmark such as symphysis pubis, umbilicus, or adherent uterus for reference, ultrasound-guided needed localization can be helpful to locate the nodule and minimize dissection.

Ecker and colleagues[22] first reported a laparoscopic approach to AWE with a focus on subfascial lesions. Melnyk and colleagues[19] further described this technique in her case series of surgically managed RME. The advantages of minimally invasive surgery, including less postoperative pain, lower infection rates, shorter hospital stay, and quicker return to normal activities, are additional benefits of laparoscopy over an abdominal approach.[33] The laparoscopic approach also provides an opportunity for the treatment of pelvic endometriosis if present and the patient is symptomatic. We suggest the following approach to surgical excision. If most of the endometriotic nodule is within the subcutaneous tissue, an abdominal approach is preferred. When the bulk of the disease is subfascial and involving the rectus body, a laparoscopic approach is most appropriate.[33] The surgical procedure is billed according to the corresponding Current Procedural Terminology codes (**Table 1**).

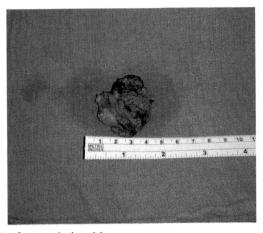

**Fig. 3.** AWE nodule after surgical excision.

| Table 1 | |
|---|---|
| Current procedural terminology codes for surgical management of abdominal wall endometriosis | |
| CPT Code | Description |
| 22902 | Excision of abdominal wall, subcutaneous, <3 cm |
| 22903 | Excision of abdominal wall, subcutaneous, 3 cm or greater |
| 22900 | Excision of abdominal wall (subfascial), <5 cm |
| 22901 | Excision of abdominal wall subfascial tumor, 5 cm or greater |

## SURGICAL TECHNIQUES
### Surgical Excision via an Abdominal Incision

The nodule is palpated and marked in the preoperative area, allowing for patient input and identification. The patient is placed in a supine position. The abdomen is prepped in the usual sterile fashion. The nodule is again palpated, and the planned incision is marked directly over the implant. A horizontal skin incision is made, approximately 1 to 2 cm larger than the size of the nodule to allow for dissection.[17] The subcutaneous layers are dissected until the nodule is identified, constantly palpating the lesion to guide dissection. Once the nodule is exposed, it is grasped with a clamp to provide elevation and countertraction. A stay suture is an alternative option for retraction. Using electrocautery, the disease is sharply dissected from the surrounding abdominal wall layers in a circumferential manner. During dissection, a curved hemostat can be helpful to delineate the fibrosis from the surrounding tissue.[19] Tactile feedback identifies the margins of the nodule, allowing for complete resection. Once the lesion is removed, the fascia is inspected. We recommend a tension-free fascial closure using delayed absorbable monofilament suture. When the fascial defect is too large for a tension-free repair, general surgery or plastic surgery should be consulted for abdominal wall reconstruction with or without mesh. The subcutaneous space is irrigated and closed if the depth of the defect is greater than 2 cm to prevent seroma and hematoma formation. Local anesthesia is infiltrated in the incision, and patients can be discharged home the same day.

### Surgical Excision via Laparoscopy

The location of the nodule is palpated and marked in the preoperative area, allowing for patient input and identification. Laparoscopic entry into the peritoneal cavity is standardly performed. A 45°-angled laparoscope improves visualization of the anterior abdominal wall. Using tactile palpation, anatomic landmarks, and knowledge from preoperative imaging, the endometriosis nodule is identified. A peritoneal incision is made with electrocautery at the site of the endometriosis nodule in the anterior abdominal wall. The incision is extended with careful avoidance of the inferior epigastric vessels and the bladder. If necessary, the space of Retzius is dissected to separate the bladder from the abdominal wall endometriosis nodule.[19] The nodule is grasped from the assistant ports, and downward traction delineates the borders (Fig. 4). Using a mixture of sharp and blunt dissection, the nodule is progressively dissected from the surrounding abdominal wall using monopolar energy or an advanced energy device. Tactile feedback delineates the fibrosis from the normal tissue in a circumferential fashion. After complete enucleation, the fascia is carefully inspected for defects. Small defects (<3 cm) are repaired with interrupted delayed absorbable sutures using a fascial closure device (Fig. 5).[19] Melnyk and colleagues[19]

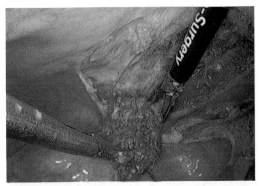

**Fig. 4.** During laparoscopic excision of AWE, downward traction on the lesion from the assistant port helps delineate the borders of the lesion to facilitate dissection.

first described repairing larger defects (>3 cm) with mesh and absorbable tacks. A multidisciplinary approach with general surgery, particularly a laparoscopic hernia specialist, is helpful for complex laparoscopic repairs and reconstruction.

### Surgical Management of Pelvic Endometriosis

Laparoscopic evaluation of the pelvis for concurrent endometriosis should be considered in patients who present with pelvic symptoms. The reported rates of coexisting pelvic endometriosis with AWE range from 5% to 34%.[4,5,14,19,34–37] Patients with AWE and no prior surgery have a higher likelihood of having pelvic endometriosis, specifically deep infiltrating disease. Marras and colleagues[4] found that patients with concurrent pelvic endometriosis were more likely to be nulliparous, present with smaller nodules, and have nodules located in the umbilicus and suprapubic region. This study also reported that AWE associated with a cesarean delivery scar is less likely to have concurrent pelvic disease.[4] Pelvic endometriosis, when present, frequently involves the bladder (**Fig. 6**). In one series, 70% of patients who underwent laparoscopic excision of RME had concurrent pelvic endometriosis with the most common location being the bladder or ureter (60%).[19] The anatomic relationship between the anterior abdominal wall and the bladder is altered with cesarean deliveries, which could represent the reason for the high incidence of genitourinary disease. Another hypothesis is

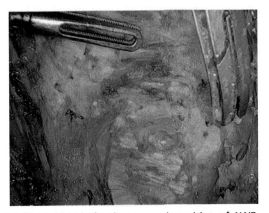

**Fig. 5.** Small fascial defect is noted after laparoscopic excision of AWE.

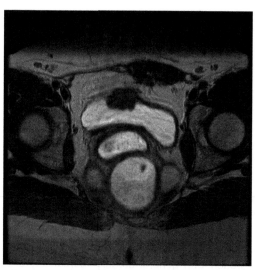

**Fig. 6.** MRI image with AWE and concurrent bladder endometriosis nodules.

that endometrial cells are seeded into the bladder when dissecting the bladder flap during a cesarean delivery. We recommend surgical exploration of the pelvis in patients with AWE who present with symptoms of endometriosis such as dyspareunia, dyschezia, and/or pelvic pain, with a heightened clinical suspicion in patients with spontaneous AWE, because their incidence of concurrent pelvic endometriosis is higher than the general population.[21]

### Treatment Outcome

Surgical management of AWE results in symptom relief with most studies reporting greater than 90% complete relief on short-term follow-up.[12,18,19,21,38] Recurrence risk ranges from 4.3% to 11%, and recurrences can be minimized by ensuring adequate margins during surgery.[4,12,21,38] Recurrences typically occur years later, and only one study demonstrated a lower recurrence rate in patients treated with hormonal medications compared with those not on suppression.[4,12,18] Malignant transformation of AWE is extremely rate with a reported incidence of 0.3% to 1%.[39] The evidence is limited to case reports, with 46 cases described in the literature. Two-thirds of malignancies are clear cell carcinoma.[3,39] Compared with benign lesions, cancerous masses are larger at diagnosis with a median diameter of 9 cm and present at a later interval, with median time of 18 years from initial surgery to diagnosis.[39,40] The clinical presentation is otherwise similar to that of benign AWE.[39–42] In cases of suspected malignancy, we recommend early referral to gynecologic oncology because these cancers are aggressive and associated with poor clinical outcomes.

### Prevention

There is no evidence that specific surgical techniques prevent incisional seeding during abdominal surgery and the subsequent development of AWE.[3] Suggested strategies include irrigation of the abdominal incision, changing gloves before fascial closure, and using fresh surgical instruments to close the fascia.[12] Although these strategies may reflect best surgical practice, there is no evidence that they will prevent the development of AWE.[3,17] Because greater than 80% of cases of AWE are associated with a cesarean delivery, preventing the primary cesarean delivery may decrease the prevalence of subsequent AWE.

## DISCUSSION

AWE is a rare form of endometriosis with which many providers are unfamiliar, resulting in a delay in diagnosis and patient suffering. Patients experience symptoms for 1 to 3 years before surgical treatment.[14,18,36] The clinical presentation of cyclic focal abdominal pain adjacent to a cesarean delivery scar is pathognomonic, yet in patients with this presentation Andres and colleagues[21] cited a preoperative clinical diagnosis of only 39%. A heightened clinical suspicion is crucial to making the diagnosis, and education should be directed to general surgeons and primary care providers, because up to 70% of patients with AWE are referred to general surgery.[21]

Experts differentiate between the 2 types of AWE based on pathogenesis and clinical presentation. The most common presentation of AWE is following major abdominal surgery, typically a cesarean delivery. Endometrial cells are iatrogenically transplanted into the surgical incision, and over time the endometriosis grows and proliferates in response to hormonal stimulation. The incidence of AWE following a cesarean delivery is 0.5% to 1% and is not related to the number of prior cesarean deliveries, timing of delivery, or reason for cesarean delivery.[3,4,22] AWE after cesarean delivery presents a singular nodule in the apices of the Pfannenstiel incision without concurrent pelvic endometriosis. Although cesarean delivery is the most common preceding surgical procedure, AWE can grow in scars from other pelvic surgeries including trocar sites from laparoscopic surgery.[14]

Spontaneous AWE that occurs in the absence of a prior surgical incision is the rarer type of AWE and most commonly presents in the groin or at the umbilicus. Endometrial cells are transplanted via lymphatic drainage from the pelvis to the groin where they implant and grow. The pathogenesis of spontaneous umbilical endometriosis is less clear and hypothesized to be secondary to vascular or lymphatic spread to the narrowest portion of the abdominal wall.[22] Ecker and colleagues[22] reported that patients presenting with no prior surgical history had higher rates of dysmenorrhea and were more likely to be nulliparous compared with AWE following cesarean delivery. Concurrent pelvic endometriosis, specifically deep infiltrating endometriosis, is more common in this population and likely contributes to the pathogenesis.

Surgical excision is standard of care for both variations of AWE, and preoperative imaging informs surgical planning. Abdominal ultrasonography is the first-line image modality to confirm the diagnosis and exclude other causes of an abdominal wall mass. MRI is recommended for patients with larger lesions and in patients in whom suspected AWE is difficult to palpate on physical examination. Surgical approach should be determined by the size, location and layers of the abdominal wall involved, and with surgeon comfort. The authors recommend a laparoscopic approach when the bulk of disease is subfascial and involving the rectus muscle. The traditional abdominal approach is preferred if the lesion is located in the subcutaneous tissue. For both surgical techniques, preoperative collaboration with a multidisciplinary team including general or plastic surgery is recommended for lesions with greater than 3 cm of fascial involvement. Two-thirds of AWE involves the fascia, and mesh is necessary in up to 10% of cases.[17] Larger size and deeper nodules invading the rectus are associated with higher rates of recurrent disease, and obtaining a 1 cm margin is the recommended practice to reduce recurrence.[17,21] Careful preoperative planning allows for complete surgical resection. Following surgery, patients have good short-term pain relief, but long-term outcomes are not published in the literature.

With the increasing rate of cesarean deliveries worldwide, the incidence of AWE will likely increase and continue to represent a diagnostic challenge for clinicians. Therefore, physician education regarding clinical presentation and management of AWE is increasingly important. The available literature is low quality, because most publications are retrospective single-institution case series and expert opinion with short-term follow-up. Andres and colleagues[21] suggest establishing a worldwide registry to improve evidence-based care of this disease. This registry would allow for prospective comparative research studies to answer important clinical questions.

## CLINICS CARE POINTS

- Prior abdominal surgery, specifically a cesarean delivery, is the largest risk factor for AWE, with 80% of cases associated with a prior surgical scar.
- The pathognomonic triad of AWE is cyclic abdominal pain, a palpable mass, and a history of abdominal surgery.
- Abdominal ultrasonography is the first-line imaging modality for AWE, with preoperative detection rates as high as 97%.
- MRI should be considered for lesions greater than 3 cm to inform surgical planning.
- Medical management with OCPs, progestins, or GnRH agonists can be considered for temporary symptom relief but will not reduce lesion size.
- Surgical excision with 1-cm margins is standard of care for treatment of AWE.
- AWE involves the fascia in two-thirds of cases, and a multidisciplinary surgical team is necessary when the fascial defect is greater than 3 cm to perform abdominal wall reconstruction with or without mesh.
- Surgical management results in symptomatic relief, with reported rates of complete relief at short term follow-up as high as greater than 90%.

## DISCLOSURE

The authors have nothing to disclose. The authors declare no financial support for this project.

## REFERENCES

1. Practice bulletin no. 114: management of endometriosis. Obstet Gynecol 2010; 116(1):223–36. https://doi.org/10.1097/AOG.0b013e3181e8b073.
2. Zondervan KT, Becker CM, Missmer SA. Endometriosis. N Engl J Med 2020; 382(13):1244–56.
3. Allen SE, Rindos NB, Mansuria S. Abdominal wall endometriosis: an update in diagnosis, perioperative considerations and management. Curr Opin Obstet Gynecol 2021;33(4):288–95.
4. Marras S, Pluchino N, Petignat P, et al. Abdominal wall endometriosis: An 11-year retrospective observational cohort study. Eur J Obstet Gynecol Reprod Biol X 2019;4:100096.
5. Blanco RG, Parithivel VS, Shah AK, et al. Abdominal wall endometriomas. Am J Surg 2003;185(6):596–8.
6. Hensen JH, Van Breda Vriesman AC, Puylaert JB. Abdominal wall endometriosis: clinical presentation and imaging features with emphasis on sonography. AJR Am J Roentgenol 2006;186(3):616–20.

7. Patterson GK, Winburn GB. Abdominal wall endometriomas: report of eight cases. Am Surg 1999;65(1):36–9.
8. Coley BD, Casola G. Incisional endometrioma involving the rectus abdominis muscle and subcutaneous tissues: CT appearance. AJR Am J Roentgenol 1993;160(3):549–50.
9. Granese R, Cucinella G, Barresi V, et al. Isolated endometriosis on the rectus abdominis muscle in women without a history of abdominal surgery: a rare and intriguing finding. J Minim Invasive Gynecol 2009;16(6):798–801.
10. Ideyi SC, Schein M, Niazi M, et al. Spontaneous endometriosis of the abdominal wall. Dig Surg 2003;20(3):246–8.
11. Tomás E, Martín A, Garfia C, et al. Abdominal wall endometriosis in absence of previous surgery. J Ultrasound Med 1999;18(5):373–4.
12. Zhang P, Sun Y, Zhang C, et al. Cesarean scar endometriosis: presentation of 198 cases and literature review. BMC Womens Health 2019;19(1):14.
13. Collins AM, Power KT, Gaughan B, et al. Abdominal wall reconstruction for a large caesarean scar endometrioma. Surgeon 2009;7(4):252–3.
14. Sumathy S, Mangalakanthi J, Purushothaman K, et al. Symptomatology and surgical perspective of scar endometriosis: a case series of 16 women. J Obstet Gynaecol India 2017;67(3):218–23.
15. Coeman V, Sciot R, Van Breuseghem I. Case report. Rectus abdominis endometriosis: a report of two cases. Br J Radiol 2005;78(925):68–71.
16. Khan Zaraq, Valentina Zanfagnin, El-Nashar Sherif A, et al. Risk factors, clinical presentation, and outcomes for abdominal wall endometriosis. J Minim Invasive Gynecol 2017;24(3):478–84.
17. Rindos NB, Mansuria S. Diagnosis and management of abdominal wall endometriosis: a systematic review and clinical recommendations. Obstet Gynecol Surv 2017;72(2):116–22.
18. Zhang J, Liu X. Clinicopathological features of endometriosis in abdominal wall–clinical analysis of 151 cases. Clin Exp Obstet Gynecol 2016;43(3):379–83.
19. Melnyk A, Foley CE, Lee TT. Endometriosis of the rectus muscle: a single center experience. J Gynecol Surg 2020;222:S818–9.
20. Giannella L, La Marca A, Ternelli G, et al. Rectus abdominis muscle endometriosis: case report and review of the literature. J Obstet Gynaecol Res 2010; 36(4):902–6.
21. Andres MP, Arcoverde FVL, Souza CCC, et al. Extrapelvic endometriosis: a systematic review. J Minim Invasive Gynecol 2020;27(2):373–89.
22. Ecker AM, Donnellan NM, Shepherd JP, et al. Abdominal wall endometriosis: 12 years of experience at a large academic institution. Am J Obstet Gynecol 2014; 211(4):363.e1–3635.
23. Haim N, Shapiro-Feinberg M, Zissin R. Incisional endometriomas: CT findings. Emerg Radiol 2005;11(3):162–3.
24. Busard MP, Mijatovic V, van Kuijk C, et al. Appearance of abdominal wall endometriosis on MR imaging. Eur Radiol 2010;20(5):1267–76.
25. Zhao X, Lang J, Leng J, et al. Abdominal wall endometriomas. Int J Gynaecol Obstet 2005;90(3):218–22.
26. Singh M, Sivanesan K, Ghani R, et al. Caesarean scar endometriosis. Arch Gynecol Obstet 2009;279(2):217–9.
27. Nissotakis C, Zouros E, Revelos K, et al. Abdominal wall endometrioma: a case report and review of the literature. AORN J 2010;91(6):730–45.

28. Wang S, Li BH, Wang JJ, et al. The safety of echo contrast-enhanced ultrasound in high-intensity focused ultrasound ablation for abdominal wall endometriosis: a retrospective study. Quant Imaging Med Surg 2021;11(5):1751–62.

29. Zhao L, Deng Y, Wei Q, et al. Comparison of ultrasound-guided high-intensity focused ultrasound ablation and surgery for abdominal wall endometriosis. Int J Hyperthermia 2018;35(1):528–33.

30. Zhu X, Chen L, Deng X, et al. A comparison between high-intensity focused ultrasound and surgical treatment for the management of abdominal wall endometriosis. BJOG 2017;124(Suppl 3):53–8.

31. Welch BT, Ehman EC, VanBuren WM, et al. Percutaneous cryoablation of abdominal wall endometriosis: the Mayo Clinic approach. Abdom Radiol (Ny) 2020;45(6):1813–7.

32. Maillot J, Brun JL, Dubuisson V, et al. Mid-term outcomes after percutaneous cryoablation of symptomatic abdominal wall endometriosis: comparison with surgery alone in a single institution. Eur Radiol 2017;27(10):4298–306.

33. Mohiuddin K, Swanson SJ. Maximizing the benefit of minimally invasive surgery. J Surg Oncol 2013;108(5):315–9.

34. Matalliotakis M, Matalliotaki C, Zervou MI, et al. Abdominal and perineal scar endometriosis: Retrospective study on 40 cases. Eur J Obstet Gynecol Reprod Biol 2020;252:225–7.

35. Cho YK, Kocol D, Harkins G, et al. An approach to abdominal-wall endometriosis: a retrospective case series. J Gynecol Surg 2020;36:1–4.

36. Ding Y, Zhu J. A retrospective review of abdominal wall endometriosis in Shanghai, China. Int J Gynaecol Obstet 2013;121(1):41–4.

37. Wolf Y, Haddad R, Werbin N, et al. Endometriosis in abdominal scars: a diagnostic pitfall. Am Surg 1996;62(12):1042–4.

38. Horton JD, Dezee KJ, Ahnfeldt EP, et al. Abdominal wall endometriosis: a surgeon's perspective and review of 445 cases. Am J Surg 2008;196(2):207–12.

39. Bedell S, Chang Z, Burt C, et al. Incisional carcinoma of mullerian origin: a case report and review of literature. Gynecol Oncol Rep 2020;33:100588.

40. Ferrandina G, Palluzzi E, Fanfani F, et al. Endometriosis-associated clear cell carcinoma arising in caesarean section scar: a case report and review of the literature. World J Surg Oncol 2016;14(1):300.

41. Paulino E, de Melo AC, da Silva VF. Endometrioid carcinoma arising from an endometriosis-associated abdominal wall scar. Am J Case Rep 2020;21:e922973.

42. Giannella L, Serri M, Maccaroni E, et al. Endometriosis-associated clear cell carcinoma of the abdominal wall after caesarean section: a case report and review of the literature. Vivo 2020;34(4):2147–52.

# Enhanced Recovery After Surgery in Minimally Invasive Gynecologic Surgery

Lisa Chao, MD*, Emily Lin, MD, Kimberly Kho, MD, MPH

## KEYWORDS

- Enhanced recovery • ERAS • Fast track • Minimally invasive gynecologic surgery
- Gynecologic surgery • Same-day discharge • Perioperative care

## KEY POINTS

- Enhanced recovery after surgery (ERAS) strategies focus on multimodal approaches to optimize patient outcomes by minimizing surgical stress with the goal of returning to normal physiologic function.
- ERAS pathways in minimally invasive gynecologic surgery have resulted in improved patient outcomes, reduced postoperative complications, increased patient satisfaction, and higher rates of same-day discharge.
- A multidisciplinary approach throughout the surgical experience and compliance with ERAS protocols are crucial for successful implementation.
- ERAS utilization can have a positive impact on health care quality and should be considered for all gynecologic surgery, including minimally invasive procedures.

## INTRODUCTION

The "enhanced recovery after surgery" (ERAS) concept allows for optimization of perioperative care through an evidence-based, multimodal approach, which has been proven to benefit the patient as well as health care systems. The underlying principle of ERAS is to optimize patient outcomes by minimizing surgical stress with the goal of returning to normal physiologic function.[1] Using minimally invasive surgery as the preferred route of surgery whenever possible is an integral component of ERAS, and is strongly associated with improved postoperative outcomes.[2] Surgical stress forces the body into a catabolic state, which results in increased cardiac demands, relative tissue hypoxia, increased insulin resistance, and altered pulmonary and gastrointestinal function.[3] ERAS protocols aim to minimize surgical stress through an integrated perioperative management plan that identifies sources of operative

Division of Gynecology, Department of Obstetrics and Gynecology, University of Texas Southwestern Medical Center, 5323 Harry Hines Boulevard, Dallas, TX 75390, USA
* Corresponding author.
*E-mail address:* Lisa.Chao@utsouthwestern.edu
Twitter: @LChaoMD (L.C.); @KimberlyKho1 (K.K.)

Obstet Gynecol Clin N Am 49 (2022) 381–395
https://doi.org/10.1016/j.ogc.2022.02.014
0889-8545/22/© 2022 Elsevier Inc. All rights reserved.

obgyn.theclinics.com

stress whose prevention decreases morbidity and enhances important metrics of surgical outcomes such as surgical site infection, length of hospital stay, and patient satisfaction. ERAS protocols have been widely adapted and modified through many surgical subspecialties including gynecologic surgery.[4-7] Although minimally invasive surgery alone has been shown to reduce postoperative pain, length of hospital stay, blood loss, and postoperative complications, using minimally invasive techniques in combination with ERAS principles generates additive benefits, allowing for improved outcomes and faster recovery.[2]

The paradigm shift from traditional perioperative care models to ERAS has revolutionized gynecologic surgery by improving clinical outcomes and enhancing the success of early discharge programs. Early or same-day discharge (SDD) after minimally invasive hysterectomy is safe and feasible, and is aligned with the aims of high-quality, cost-effective care. Borrowing from early successes in the colorectal surgery literature, ERAS protocols have been successfully implemented in gynecologic oncology. An increasing number of urogynecologic and minimally invasive gynecologic surgeons have also incorporated ERAS pathways into their standard perioperative care for patients undergoing benign procedures including hysterectomy, myomectomy, adnexal surgery, and pelvic organ prolapse surgeries.[8-15] The benefits of achieving higher quality surgical care with better surgical outcomes, lower health-related costs, and improved patient experience with minimally invasive gynecologic surgery (MIGS) are further enhanced with the application of ERAS.[16] This article reviews the key components of ERAS and its impact in MIGS.

## ENHANCED RECOVERY AFTER SURGERY COMPONENTS

ERAS principles can be divided into 3 segments of patient care: preoperative, intraoperative, and postoperative. Although ERAS utilization has been documented in the general gynecologic literature, its concepts are equally applicable to MIGS with its guidelines applied across the perioperative period to mitigate the physiologic stress response to surgery and promote recovery.[16]

## PREOPERATIVE CONSIDERATIONS

Preoperative enhanced recovery begins with the identification of patient comorbidities for the selection of appropriate surgical candidates, education and counseling, and management of expectations. A multidisciplinary approach to patient education is associated with decreased postoperative complications, superior pain control, and decreased recovery time.[17] The team may consist of providers including anesthesiologists, nursing staff, pharmacists, and patient educators whose goal is to encourage patients to be active participants in their recovery.[18] Establishing expectations, such as anticipation about hospital length of stay (LOS) and discharge criteria, is key to patient success. This can be performed through various modalities including counseling patients in an outpatient setting or developing educational materials using handouts, pamphlets, or online videos.[18]

Other important elements involve preoperative carbohydrate loading, cessation of alcohol and tobacco use, and avoidance of preoperative starvation by allowing clear liquids up to 2 hours before surgery. Fasting is known to be associated with impaired glucose metabolism and increased insulin resistance and therefore not recommended.[19] ERAS protocols support the administration of oral carbohydrate drinks preoperatively as they may reverse some effects of the preoperative fasting period, prevent insulin resistance and hyperglycemia, and lead to a shorter hospital LOS.[20] A summary of preoperative counseling and patient education recommendations can be seen in **Table 1**.

Optimization of modifiable risk factors such as preoperative anemia and hyperglycemia before elective gynecologic surgery should be performed to minimize risks, complications, and mortality.[16] Preoperative anemia is a strong predictor of perioperative blood transfusion and is associated with increased incidence of alloimmune sensitization, surgical site infection, and prolonged hospitalization.[21,22] Uncontrolled

**Table 1**
**Key components for preoperative counseling and patient education**

| Preoperative Considerations: Counseling and Education | |
|---|---|
| Initial Assessment and Patient Optimization | History and physical examination<br>Screen for and optimize chronic conditions (including diabetes, anemia, etc)<br>Screen for tobacco, alcohol use; counsel patients on cessation for 4–6 wk before surgery<br>Assess for malnutrition and need for weight loss; consider referral to dietitian or nutritional supplementation before surgery<br>Encourage 30 min of walking daily until surgery<br>Assess risk for postoperative nausea and vomiting using simplified Apfel criteria[a] |
| Diet Instructions | Encourage protein and CHO-rich foods for 1 wk preceding surgery<br>Allow clear liquids, ideally 50-g CHO-rich beverage, until 2 h before surgery<br>Clear liquids: water, black coffee, clear tea, carbonated beverages, fruit juice without pulp, Gatorade<br>For patients with diabetes: avoid sugar-containing liquids unless hypoglycemic<br>Routine mechanical bowel preparation is not recommended |
| Setting Expectations and Patient Education | Written information provided on ERAS pathway including diet/NPO instructions (as above), preoperative shower instructions, and review of discharge medications<br>Send prescriptions for discharge medications preoperatively<br>Review plan for same-day discharge if eligible or expected length of stay if planned admission<br>Review expected postoperative pain course, bowel and bladder function changes, vaginal bleeding<br>Review plan for postoperative urinary retention<br>Review postoperative activity recommendations |
| Providing Reassurance | Preoperative phone call placed the day before surgery by RN to rereview instructions with patient<br>Ensure patients know how to contact providers during business hours and after-hours |

*Abbreviations:* CHO, carbohydrate; NPO, nil per os, or nothing by mouth; PONV, postoperative nausea and vomiting; RN, registered nurse.
[a] Apfel criteria: female gender, nonsmoker, history of PONV, postoperative opioid use -> 0 to 1 risk factors is LOW, 2 risk factors is MEDIUM, ≥3 risk factors is HIGH.

diabetes in patients undergoing gynecologic surgery is associated with increased risk of needing prolonged postoperative ventilation and critical care, longer hospital stays, and complications.[16] The AAGL Task Force, composed of US and Canadian gynecologic surgery experts on ERAS subject matter, recommends targeting hemoglobin (Hgb) level thresholds $\geq$12 g/dL for elective surgery and postponing patients with glycated Hgb levels $\geq$8.5%.[16]

Additional preoperative elements include avoidance of bowel preparations, multimodal preemptive analgesia, and postoperative nausea prophylaxis.[18] A meta-analysis performed by Arnold and colleagues revealed no evidence of benefit of mechanical bowel preparation in gynecologic surgery and therefore bowel preparations are not routinely incorporated in ERAS protocols.[23] The goal of preemptive analgesia in ERAS pathways is to prevent the activation of pain receptors during surgery. Medications with varying mechanisms of action, such as acetaminophen and COX-2 inhibitors are given before skin incision with the aim to reduce postoperative narcotic pain medication requirements. Multimodal analgesic regimens have relied on nonopioid pharmacologic agents, use of locoregional anesthetics, and adjunct therapies such as dexamethasone.[16] Preoperative dexamethasone has analgesic properties and can serve as both nausea and pain prophylaxis.[24] Regional analgesia, such as the use of thoracic epidural analgesia (TEA), is commonly a part of ERAS pathways in colorectal and other types of open surgery to mitigate postoperative pain.[25] Although the use of TEA has been associated with decreased opioid use, its benefit in minimally invasive gynecologic procedures remains unclear given that patients undergoing laparoscopic or robotic procedures already have reduced pain and a shorter length of hospital stay. Pain prevention procedures such as port-site infiltration with short-acting local anesthetic agents and regional blocks such as the transversus abdominis plane (TAP) blocks and paracervical blocks have also been used with mixed results.[16]

Postoperative nausea prophylaxis given preoperatively is also a significant component of ERAS protocols. Well-known risk factors for postoperative nausea and vomiting (PONV) include gynecologic surgery, the female gender, and minimally invasive surgery.[26] Where PONV can lead to patient dissatisfaction, prolonged hospital LOS, and unplanned admissions/readmissions, ERAS pathways incorporate the use of at least 2 antiemetic agents from different classes as a preventative measure since the effect of antiemetics acting on different receptors are additive and combination therapy is preferable to a single drug.[26] In addition, the use of transdermal scopolamine patches can have an additive benefit along with the use of antiemetic medications in the prevention of PONV.[18] Validated scoring systems such as the Apfel risk score have been used to predict the risk of PONV and the use of various preemptive prophylaxis agents can be determined based on risk factors.[27] A sample ERAS protocol, including preoperative medications, can be seen in **Table 2**.

## INTRAOPERATIVE CONSIDERATIONS

Intraoperative enhanced recovery pathways hinge on collaboration between the surgical service and anesthesia providers in prevention of PONV, fluid and temperature management, and preemptive analgesia. Intraoperative anesthesia focuses on the use of short-acting agents and regional blocks, which have been associated with decreased opioid use intraoperatively (see **Table 2**).[18] ERAS protocols typically call for the use of total intravenous anesthesia, which can involve the use of propofol infusion instead of volatile anesthetics or nitrous oxide to reduce PONV.[26] Fluid restriction and maintenance of euvolemia by avoiding intraoperative fluid overload reduce postoperative complications, expedite return of bowel function, decrease PONV, and

**Table 2**
**Sample enhanced recovery after surgery protocol**

| | Day of Surgery |
|---|---|
| Preoperative Recommendations and Medications | No routine preoperative fluid administration<br>No routine IV opioid premedication<br>Multimodal analgesia:<br>    Ibuprofen, 600 mg; or celecoxib, 400 mg po (200 mg if age >65 y<br>       and contraindicated if sulfa allergy) if GFR $\geq$30<br>    Acetaminophen, 1000 mg po (omit if hepatic dysfunction)<br>Postoperative nausea and vomiting (PONV) prophylaxis:<br>    Dexamethasone, 8 mg IV (omit for patients with poorly<br>       controlled diabetes); or perphenazine, 8 mg po<br>    Scopolamine patch for high-risk PONV if age < 65 yo<br>DVT prophylaxis:<br>    Routine use of sequential compression devices<br>    Preoperative subcutaneous heparin 5000u when indicated |
| Intraoperative Recommendations | Antibiotic prophylaxis if indicated<br>Induction of anesthesia:<br>    Propofol, 1-2 mg/kg IV<br>    Ketamine, 20 mg IV<br>    Lidocaine, 100–200 mg IV bolus<br>    Muscle relaxant (no opioids)<br>Maintenance of anesthesia:<br>    Propofol TIVA—no nitrous oxide or remifentanil<br>    Ketamine, 10 mg q 1 hour following initial bolus<br>    Lidocaine, 100 mg IV bolus q 1 hour<br>    Magnesium, 2g IV over 1 h (no bolus)<br>Temperature management: fluid warmer, underbody warming<br>    blanket, Bair Hugger<br>Fluid management:<br>    Maintain euvolemia, avoid excess positive fluid balance<br>    Avoid normal saline in favor of balanced crystalloid<br>    (eg, PlasmaLyte, Lactated Ringers)<br>    IV boluses of 200–300 mL crystalloid for MAP < 60 mm Hg or<br>    30% of baseline<br>Emergence:<br>    Propofol titration<br>    Ondansetron, 4 mg IV<br>    Ketorolac, 15 mg IV<br>Local infiltration of incision sites by surgeons<br>Consider TAP block if indicated |
| Postoperative Recovery Unit Recommendations | IV -> po opioids for breakthrough pain; avoid PCA<br>Start ice chips and sips of clear liquids as tolerated<br>IV fluids at 40 mL/h until tolerating po |
| Discharge Medications | Acetaminophen, 650 mg q 6 hours po<br>Ibuprofen, 600 mg q 6 hours po (can alternate with<br>    acetaminophen)<br>Oxycodone, 5 mg q 6 hours po as needed for breakthrough pain<br>Ondansetron, 8 mg po q 8 hours × 24 h if high-risk for PONV<br>Senna, 8.6 mg po daily until regular bowel movements have<br>    returned<br>Enoxaparin if indicated<br>Hormone replacement therapy if indicated |

*(continued on next page)*

| Table 2 (continued) | |
| --- | --- |
| | **Day of Surgery** |
| Discharge Criteria | Spontaneous voiding trial completed or Foley catheter placed for urinary retention<br>Tolerating po without nausea or emesis<br>Pain controlled (pain score < 5)<br>Independently ambulating |

*Abbreviations:* DVT, deep vein thrombosis; GFR, glomerular filtration rate; IV, intravenous; MAP, mean arterial pressure; PCA, patient-controlled analgesia; po, per os, or by mouth; PONV, postoperative nausea and vomiting; TIVA, total intravenous anesthesia.

shorten hospital LOS.[18] Emphasis is placed on minimizing the use of crystalloids and increasing colloid use to achieve euvolemia and avoid fluid overload.[28] Fluid overload can lead to electrolyte abnormalities, peripheral soft tissue edema that can impair early mobility, and small bowel edema that can result in delayed return of bowel function.[18]

Intraoperative body core temperatures below 36°C have been associated with coagulopathy, increased risk of bleeding, impaired drug metabolism, impaired oxygen transportation, cardiac morbidity, and infectious wound morbidity.[18] Thus, supporting body temperature with a Bair Hugger and warmed intravenous fluids maintains normothermia, which is associated with improved patient outcomes.[29,30] In addition, routine nasogastric tube placement in both benign and gynecologic oncology is discouraged because avoiding its use has resulted in earlier return of bowel function.[31] However, the avoidance of routine nasogastric or orogastric tube placement may not always apply to minimally invasive gynecologic procedures, as it is necessary to decompress the stomach to facilitate safer trocar placement and should be removed upon reversal of anesthesia.

## POSTOPERATIVE CONSIDERATIONS

The optimal analgesic regimen for surgery should provide adequate pain relief, allow for early mobilization and early return of bowel function, and minimize complications.[32] Multimodal analgesia aims to avoid or minimize the use of opioids and their side effects, a concept that is paramount in enhanced recovery pathways (see **Table 2**).[33] Randomized controlled trials in gynecologic literature demonstrate that early postoperative feeding results in prompt return of bowel function and shorter length of hospital stay with no change in postoperative complications.[18] Postoperative enhanced recovery pathways, therefore, include early feeding while maintaining the concept of euvolemia. Minimizing intravenous hydration is important because overhydrating has been associated with poor postoperative outcomes such as delayed return of bowel function and prolonged LOS.[18] Postoperative bowel regimens are also important for patients undergoing MIGS, particularly pelvic floor reconstructive procedures as bowel regimens with senna have been shown to decrease time to first bowel movement.[34] ERAS protocols also support the removal of urinary catheters within 24 hours of surgery, even immediately following completion of minimally invasive procedures planned for early discharge.

Early mobilization and multimodal pharmacologic analgesia are paramount in ERAS protocols. The efficacy of multimodal pharmacologic analgesia relies on the synergistic effect of 2 or more medications, which can include non–opiate-containing drugs along with nonsteroidal anti-inflammatory drugs (NSAIDs) or COX-2 inhibitors.[18] Many pathways incorporate the use of ketorolac in the postoperative period as it provides adequate pain relief, equivalent to the effect of opioids.[35] Acetaminophen is an essential part of multimodal analgesia, with an intravenous formulation available. Scheduled non-narcotic agents can also be used to minimize narcotic consumption. These can include gabapentin or tramadol, which can also be used as a substitute for NSAIDs.[33] Lastly, socio-domestic factors, such as support at home, including dependent care needs, need to be discussed with the patient preoperatively as part of discharge planning to avoid impedance of early discharge.[18] A sample ERAS protocol illustrating postoperative medications and recommendations can be seen in **Table 2**.

## ENHANCED RECOVERY AFTER SURGERY IMPACT ON MINIMALLY INVASIVE GYNECOLOGIC SURGERY OUTCOMES
### Length of Stay

ERAS principles have been proven to reduce the length of hospital stay without increasing complications, mortality, or readmission rates in open gynecologic procedures.[36] Early or SDD is often a desired outcome in MIGS not typically seen in open abdominal gynecologic surgery. Various groups in diverse practice settings have published on the use of ERAS protocols with MIGS and show consistent results—high rates of SDD after minimally invasive hysterectomy (including vaginal, laparoscopic, and robotic-assisted laparoscopic approaches) without increase in readmission rates.[15,37–40] Yoong and colleagues reported that the median LOS among those who had vaginal hysterectomies was reduced from 45.5 to 22 hours with implementation of ERAS and the rate of discharge within 24 hours from surgery similarly increased from 15.6% to 78%.[37] Similar results with reduced LOS and increase in SDD rates have also been demonstrated in laparoscopic nonhysterectomy gynecologic surgeries and pelvic reconstructive procedures.[12,41] Peters and colleagues reported SDD rates increased by 9.4% ($P = .001$) with ERAS pathway implementation in women undergoing laparoscopic minimally invasive nonhysterectomy gynecologic procedures where 65% of the patients underwent procedures for endometriosis or chronic pelvic pain. The driving factor behind lower unplanned admissions were reductions in postoperative pain and nausea/vomiting with the implementation of ERAS.[12] Factors that may predispose patients to a longer LOS despite the implementation of ERAS pathways include increased operative time, time of case in the day, laparoscopic versus robotic approach, estimated blood loss, prior pelvic surgery, increasing body mass index (BMI), greater than 6 hours from last oral intake, American Society of Anesthesiologists (ASA) classification, age, and race.[13,42] Consideration of these factors may improve the success of SDD and reduce LOS. **Table 3** illustrates key criteria for determining patients' eligibility for SDD as well as factors to consider for patients that may require overnight admission.

### Postoperative Pain and Narcotic Use

Pain control can be a barrier to discharge and poor pain control is associated with a delay in return to routine activity. Although studies involving laparotomy and abdominal hysterectomies with the implementation of ERAS have shown significant reduction in postoperative narcotic use, the results in minimally invasive and vaginal surgery groups with the use of multimodal analgesia are similar with a higher drop in postoperative narcotic use without impact on pain scores.[1,9,38,43] A systematic review of preemptive analgesia in MIGS supports the use of port-site infiltration with short-acting local anesthetic agents as it has minimal risk, low cost, and has been shown to decrease pain

**Table 3**
**Criteria for same-day discharge eligibility and criteria to consider for overnight admission**

| Criteria for Same-Day Discharge | |
| --- | --- |
| Surgical Factors | Surgery ends before 6:00 PM |
| | No intraoperative complications (eg, expected EBL) |
| Patient Factors | Vital signs within normal range for patient including oxygen saturation > 92% |
| | No fever |
| | Baseline mental status and conversant |
| | Adequate pain control (pain score $\leq$ 4) |
| | Tolerating po without ongoing nausea or emesis |
| | Ambulating independently |
| | Passed spontaneous voiding trial or Foley catheter has been placed |
| **Criteria to Consider for Overnight Admission** | |
| Medical Factors | ASA score $\geq$3 |
| | Prior anesthesia complications |
| | History of obstructive sleep apnea |
| | Poorly controlled respiratory disease (eg, asthma, COPD) |
| | Therapeutically anticoagulated |
| | T1DM or poorly controlled T2DM |
| | History of arrhythmia, congestive heart failure, pacemaker/AICD, or hypertension (on >3 medications) |
| | Advanced kidney disease (GFR < 30 or on dialysis) |
| | Cirrhosis or daily alcohol consumption > 2 drinks |
| Sociodemographic Factors | Lack of social network: no relative or friend who can help provide care within the first 24 h of discharge |
| | Lives far from hospital (>60 miles) |
| | Age $\geq$80 y |
| | Impaired baseline cognition |
| | Impaired baseline mobility (ECOG performance status $\geq$2) |

*Abbreviations:* AICD, acute implantable cardioverter-defibrillator; COPD, chronic obstructive pulmonary disease; EBL, estimated blood loss; ECOG, Eastern Cooperative Oncology Group; GFR, glomerular filtration rate; po, per os, or by mouth; T1DM, type 1 diabetes mellitus; T2DM, type 2 diabetes mellitus.

*Adapted from* Stone R, Carey E, Fader AN, et al. Enhanced recovery and surgical optimization protocol for minimally invasive gynecologic surgery: an AAGL white paper. J Minim Invasive Gynecol. 2021;28(2):179-203; with permission.

perception among patients in the immediate postoperative period. This can be an adjunct to other ERAS interventions; however, data are lacking on whether preincision or preclosure incision blocks significantly decrease postoperative analgesic requirements.[44] In a prospective randomized controlled trial of women undergoing minimally invasive myomectomy, Xiromeritis and colleagues demonstrated that the use of multimodal anesthesia compared with traditional protocols with no preemptive or intraoperative medication resulted in lower pain scores.[45] Peters and colleagues reported a significant reduction of 64% ($P$ < .001) in total perioperative narcotic medication use in the ERAS cohort compared with conventional perioperative care in patients undergoing laparoscopic minimally invasive nonhysterectomy gynecologic procedures with also significantly lower postanesthesia care unit (PACU) pain scores at hours 2 and 3 ($P$ < .001).[12] In summary, implementation of multimodal analgesia is known to decrease narcotic use postoperatively without increasing pain scores.

## Bowel Function and Postoperative Nausea and Vomiting

Efforts to address and prevent PONV in the postoperative setting is a strong focus in ERAS pathways in MIGS as it can affect up to 70% of patients.[26] PONV is associated with significant patient dissatisfaction, longer stays in the PACU, unanticipated hospital admission, and increased health care costs.[46] The use of preoperative dexamethasone has been shown to enhance the quality of recovery while reducing nausea, pain, and fatigue and is often used with other antiemetics because of its synergistic effects for nausea and pain prophylaxis.[24,47] As a result, dexamethasone is often included in ERAS protocols. There are few studies in MIGS investigating the return of bowel function and PONV as primary outcomes. In a double-blinded randomized controlled trial comparing the use of preoperative dexamethasone versus placebo in women undergoing vaginal reconstructive surgery, Pauls and colleagues reported less nausea and vomiting, decreased need for rescue postoperative antiemetics, and lower PONV intensity and visual analog scale scores with the use of dexamethasone. In patients undergoing laparoscopic nonhysterectomy gynecologic surgeries, Peters and colleagues reported positive effects of ERAS institution on PONV.[12] Higher preoperative antiemetic administration in the ERAS group resulted in a 57% reduction in PONV medication usage in the PACU ($P < .001$) when compared with the conventional perioperative group. Furthermore, PONV was also a driving factor for unanticipated admission. This highlights the importance of preemptive administration of antiemetics preoperatively to maximize the success of outpatient surgery in MIGS.

## Complications

The advantages of MIGS include reduced postoperative complications—fewer surgical site infections, less postoperative pain, shorter hospital stay, faster recovery time, reduced blood loss and need for analgesics, and lower cost.[33,48] Reported complications rates have varied in published studies, ranging from 4.4% to 25% with the majority being minor complications.[42] Risk factors that lead to complications include BMI, estimated blood loss, case type, LOS, and length of surgery.[42,49] The implementation of ERAS among patients undergoing MIGS (robotic, laparoscopic, or vaginal surgery) compared with a control group have shown no significant changes in complication rates.[1,9,12,40,41,50] Modesitt and colleagues reported a decrease in bleeding and transfusion after ERAS implementation compared with a control group in major minimally invasive gynecologic procedures (28.1% compared with 6.5%, $P = .004$) with no differences in overall complications. Studies in pelvic reconstructive surgery, minimally invasive gynecologic oncologic surgeries, and minimally invasive nonhysterectomy gynecologic procedures have demonstrated similar results when compared with a control group—no changes in 30-day postoperative complications or morbidity with the implementation of ERAS.[12,41,51] The various components of ERAS all have a significant positive impact on patient outcomes across multiple perioperative parameters without increasing complication rates or affecting 30-day morbidity. This impact in MIGS is consistent with what has been seen across other surgical specialties.[52–55]

## Rates of Admission/Readmission

Although SDD is often a desired goal of MIGS, there is no consensus on the eligibility criteria for SDD. Preoperative factors associated with increased 30-day readmissions and therefore should not be eligible for SDD include patients with poorly controlled medical comorbidities, patients requiring therapeutic anticoagulation, and those without social support in the first 24 hours after discharge.[16] Relative contraindications to SDD include patients with advanced age ($\geq$80 years), history of stroke, morbid obesity (BMI > 50 kg/m$^2$), and obstructive sleep apnea.[16] Not only do patients have to be appropriately selected to ensure the success of ERAS pathways, but compliance to protocol guidelines is paramount to achieve maximum benefit and minimize admission and readmission rates. The 3 most common indications for admission are pain, nausea, and urinary retention. Successful protocols have highlighted pain and nausea prophylaxis and enabled discharge with urinary catheters or intermittent self-catheterization.[16] Keil and colleagues reported predictors of admission after laparoscopic hysterectomy under an ERAS pathway to be increased ASA status, being African American, and increased length of procedure. There were no significant differences in the incidence of readmissions within 90 days between those discharged same-day or admitted.[13] Further studies have shown that readmission rates for benign MIGS were between 0% and 7% where an ERAS protocol was implemented, which was not different from non-ERAS controls.[42] Several studies have also reported no differences in readmission rates for patients undergoing vaginal hysterectomies or pelvic reconstructive surgeries with and without ERAS implementation.[37,41,56] Rates of readmission for laparoscopic hysterectomy and nonhysterectomy gynecologic procedures were similar as well in both groups and ranged from 0% to 7%.[13,15,39,50,57,58] Increases in SDD with ERAS implementation have consistently shown improved perioperative outcomes in MIGS without affecting rates of readmission.

### Patient Satisfaction

In general, ERAS implementation in MIGS is met with high patient satisfaction. Trowbridge and colleagues reported that patients who underwent an enhanced recovery pathway after pelvic reconstructive surgery were satisfied with the overall hospital environment ($P = .04$), overall transition of care from the hospital to home ($P = .003$), more likely to report their pain was well-controlled ($P = .0007$), and that they had a good understanding of managing their health after discharge ($P = .0001$).[41] Modesitt and colleagues also showed a marked improvement on focus questions regarding pain control ($P < .001$), nurses keeping patients informed ($P < .001$), and staff teamwork with ERAS implementation in major gynecologic surgeries.[9] de Lapasse evaluated patient satisfaction after laparoscopic hysterectomy using a fast-track protocol and reported that 97% of patients were satisfied with the procedure and would recommend it to others.[57] Improved communication with patients and control of postoperative pain correlates with high patient satisfaction as demonstrated by ERAS protocols.

### Cost-Effectiveness

Enhanced recovery pathways can provide cost savings despite known initial implementation expenses. Yoong and colleagues and Relph and colleagues demonstrate an overall median decrease in cost per patient undergoing vaginal hysterectomy following the use of an ERAS pathway by 9.25% (£106.30/$159.45) and 12.7% (£164.86), respectively.[37,56] Both studies attribute most of the cost savings to the drastic decrease in LOS (51.6% and 45.2% reduction, respectively), despite additional increased overhead expenses required for ERAS implementation. These cost savings have been shown to be more pronounced with minimally invasive procedures. Rhou and colleagues reported a total lower cost for fast-track laparoscopic hysterectomy when compared with fast-track total abdominal hysterectomy ($P < .0001$).[59] Most of the cost savings was seen in postoperative costs ($P < .0001$), again likely related to the known decreased LOS associated with both ERAS pathways and minimally invasive surgeries. These data highlight the positive financial and economic benefits of implementing an enhanced recovery pathway, supporting their use across hospital systems, and furthermore reiterates the importance of concomitant use of minimally invasive surgical techniques.

## SUMMARY

ERAS pathways have revolutionized perioperative care for patients undergoing gynecologic surgery. Minimally invasive surgery is seen as a significant and integral component of any ERAS protocol as it has been shown to improve outcomes both separately from, and as a part of ERAS strategies. These results rely on a comprehensive approach to teamwork, emphasis on optimization, adherence and compliance to protocols, and support of data-driven change and improvement. Implementation of ERAS practices in MIGS have shown significant positive impacts such as reduction in length of hospital stay, improved patient satisfaction, decreased administration of opioids without an increase in complications, readmissions, or total hospital costs. Enhanced recovery pathways should be the standard of care in minimally invasive gynecologic procedures as it allows for high-quality patient care at minimal cost.

## CLINICS CARE POINTS

- The underlying principle of ERAS strategies is to optimize patient outcomes by minimizing surgical stress with the goal of returning to normal physiologic function.
- Using minimally invasive surgery as the preferred route of surgery whenever possible is an integral component to ERAS and is strongly associated with improved postoperative outcomes.
- Optimization of modifiable risk factors such as preoperative anemia and hyperglycemia before elective gynecologic surgery should be performed to minimize risks, complications, and mortality. The AAGL ERAS Task Force recommends targeting hemoglobin (Hgb) level thresholds $\geq 12$ g/dL for elective surgery and postponing patients with glycated Hgb levels $\geq 8.5\%$.
- Multimodal analgesia aims to avoid or minimize the use of opioids and their side effects and can include port-site infiltration of analgesics, TAP blocks, as well as NSAIDs, COX-2 inhibitors, acetaminophen, and gabapentin.
- Efforts to address and prevent postoperative nausea and vomiting (PONV) with identification of high-risk patients, and preemptive use of dexamethasone and scopolamine patches, as well as various antiemetic agents.
- Successful implementation of ERAS pathways can improve patient outcomes, increase patient satisfaction, shorten hospital length of stay, and decrease health care costs.

## DISCLOSURE

The authors have nothing to disclose.

## REFERENCES

1. Kalogera E, Bakkum-Gamez JN, Jankowski CJ, et al. Enhanced recovery in gynecologic surgery. Obstet Gynecol 2013;122(2 Pt 1):319–28.
2. Abeles A, Kwasnicki RM, Darzi A. Enhanced recovery after surgery: current research insights and future direction. World J Gastrointest Surg 2017;9(2):37–45.
3. Kehlet H, Wilmore DW. Evidence-based surgical care and the evolution of fast-track surgery. Ann Surg 2008;248(2):189–98.

4. Ljungqvist O, Scott M, Fearon KC. Enhanced recovery after surgery: a review. JAMA Surg 2017;152(3):292–8.

5. Carey ET, Moulder JK. Perioperative management and implementation of enhanced recovery programs in gynecologic surgery for benign indications. Obstet Gynecol 2018;132(1):137–46.

6. Nelson G, Kalogera E, Dowdy SC. Enhanced recovery pathways in gynecologic oncology. Gynecol Oncol 2014;135(3):586–94.

7. Trowbridge ER, Dreisbach CN, Sarosiek BM, et al. Review of enhanced recovery programs in benign gynecologic surgery. Int Urogynecol J 2018;29(1):3–11.

8. Carter-Brooks CM, Du AL, Ruppert KM, et al. Implementation of a urogynecology-specific enhanced recovery after surgery (ERAS) pathway. Am J Obstet Gynecol 2018;219(5):e491–5.

9. Modesitt SC, Sarosiek BM, Trowbridge ER, et al. Enhanced recovery implementation in major gynecologic surgeries: effect of care standardization. Obstet Gynecol 2016;128(3):457–66.

10. Nelson G, Altman AD, Nick A, et al. Guidelines for postoperative care in gynecologic/oncology surgery: enhanced recovery after surgery (ERAS(R)) society recommendations–Part II. Gynecol Oncol 2016;140(2):323–32.

11. Nelson G, Altman AD, Nick A, et al. Guidelines for pre- and intra-operative care in gynecologic/oncology surgery: enhanced recovery after surgery (ERAS(R)) society recommendations–Part I. Gynecol Oncol 2016;140(2):313–22.

12. Peters A, Siripong N, Wang L, et al. Enhanced recovery after surgery outcomes in minimally invasive nonhysterectomy gynecologic procedures. Am J Obstet Gynecol 2020;223(2):234.e1–8.

13. Keil DS, Schiff LD, Carey ET, et al. Predictors of admission after the implementation of an enhanced recovery after surgery pathway for minimally invasive gynecologic surgery. Anesth Analg 2019;129(3):776–83.

14. Lee J, Asher V, Nair A, et al. Comparing the experience of enhanced recovery programme for gynaecological patients undergoing laparoscopic versus open gynaecological surgery: a prospective study. Perioper Med (Lond) 2018;7:15.

15. Minig L, Chuang L, Patrono MG, et al. Clinical outcomes after fast-track care in women undergoing laparoscopic hysterectomy. Int J Gynaecol Obstet 2015; 131(3):301–4.

16. Stone R, Carey E, Fader AN, et al. Enhanced recovery and surgical optimization protocol for minimally invasive gynecologic surgery: an AAGL white paper. J Minim Invasive Gynecol 2021;28(2):179–203.

17. Halaszynski TM, Juda R, Silverman DG. Optimizing postoperative outcomes with efficient preoperative assessment and management. Crit Care Med 2004;32(4 Suppl):S76–86.

18. Kalogera E, Dowdy SC. Enhanced recovery pathway in gynecologic surgery: improving outcomes through evidence-based medicine. Obstet Gynecol Clin North Am 2016;43(3):551–73.

19. Svanfeldt M, Thorell A, Brismar K, et al. Effects of 3 days of "postoperative" low caloric feeding with or without bed rest on insulin sensitivity in healthy subjects. Clin Nutr 2003;22(1):31–8.

20. Mathur S, Plank LD, McCall JL, et al. Randomized controlled trial of preoperative oral carbohydrate treatment in major abdominal surgery. Br J Surg 2010;97(4): 485–94.

21. Clevenger B, Mallett SV, Klein AA, et al. Patient blood management to reduce surgical risk. Br J Surg 2015;102(11):1325–37 ; discussion 1324.

22. Zwingerman R, Jain V, Hannon J, et al. Alloimmune red blood cell antibodies: prevalence and pathogenicity in a canadian prenatal population. J Obstet Gynaecol Can 2015;37(9):784–90.
23. Arnold A, Aitchison LP, Abbott J. Preoperative mechanical bowel preparation for abdominal, laparoscopic, and vaginal surgery: a systematic review. J Minim Invasive Gynecol 2015;22(5):737–52.
24. Blanton E, Lamvu G, Patanwala I, et al. Non-opioid pain management in benign minimally invasive hysterectomy: a systematic review. Am J Obstet Gynecol 2017;216(6):557–67.
25. Nygren J, Thacker J, Carli F, et al. Guidelines for perioperative care in elective rectal/pelvic surgery: enhanced recovery after surgery (ERAS((R))) society recommendations. World J Surg 2013;37(2):285–305.
26. Apfel CC, Heidrich FM, Jukar-Rao S, et al. Evidence-based analysis of risk factors for postoperative nausea and vomiting. Br J Anaesth 2012;109(5):742–53.
27. Apfel CC, Laara E, Koivuranta M, et al. A simplified risk score for predicting postoperative nausea and vomiting: conclusions from cross-validations between two centers. Anesthesiology 1999;91(3):693–700.
28. Rahbari NN, Zimmermann JB, Schmidt T, et al. Meta-analysis of standard, restrictive and supplemental fluid administration in colorectal surgery. Br J Surg 2009; 96(4):331–41.
29. Galvao CM, Marck PB, Sawada NO, et al. A systematic review of the effectiveness of cutaneous warming systems to prevent hypothermia. J Clin Nurs 2009; 18(5):627–36.
30. Perez-Protto S, Sessler DI, Reynolds LF, et al. Circulating-water garment or the combination of a circulating-water mattress and forced-air cover to maintain core temperature during major upper-abdominal surgery. Br J Anaesth 2010; 105(4):466–70.
31. Nelson R, Edwards S, Tse B. Prophylactic nasogastric decompression after abdominal surgery. Cochrane Database Syst Rev 2007;3:CD004929.
32. Veenhof AA, Vlug MS, van der Pas MH, et al. Surgical stress response and postoperative immune function after laparoscopy or open surgery with fast track or standard perioperative care: a randomized trial. Ann Surg 2012;255(2):216–21.
33. Gustafsson UO, Scott MJ, Schwenk W, et al. Guidelines for perioperative care in elective colonic surgery: Enhanced Recovery After Surgery (ERAS((R))) Society recommendations. World J Surg 2013;37(2):259–84.
34. Patel M, Schimpf MO, O'Sullivan DM, et al. The use of senna with docusate for postoperative constipation after pelvic reconstructive surgery: a randomized, double-blind, placebo-controlled trial. Am J Obstet Gynecol 2010;202(5):479 e471–475.
35. Gobble RM, Hoang HLT, Kachniarz B, et al. Ketorolac does not increase perioperative bleeding: a meta-analysis of randomized controlled trials. Plast Reconstr Surg 2014;133(3):741–55.
36. de Groot JJ, Ament SM, Maessen JM, et al. Enhanced recovery pathways in abdominal gynecologic surgery: a systematic review and meta-analysis. Acta Obstet Gynecol Scand 2016;95(4):382–95.
37. Yoong W, Sivashanmugarajan V, Relph S, et al. Can enhanced recovery pathways improve outcomes of vaginal hysterectomy? cohort control study. J Minim Invasive Gynecol 2014;21(1):83–9.
38. Chapman JS, Roddy E, Ueda S, et al. Enhanced recovery pathways for improving outcomes after minimally invasive gynecologic oncology surgery. Obstet Gynecol 2016;128(1):138–44.

39. Lee SJ, Calderon B, Gardner GJ, et al. The feasibility and safety of same-day discharge after robotic-assisted hysterectomy alone or with other procedures for benign and malignant indications. Gynecol Oncol 2014;133(3):552–5.

40. Lambaudie E, de Nonneville A, Brun C, et al. Enhanced recovery after surgery program in gynaecologic oncological surgery in a minimally invasive techniques expert center. BMC Surg 2017;17(1):136.

41. Trowbridge ER, Evans SL, Sarosiek BM, et al. Enhanced recovery program for minimally invasive and vaginal urogynecologic surgery. Int Urogynecol J 2019; 30(2):313–21.

42. Scheib SA, Thomassee M, Kenner JL. Enhanced recovery after surgery in gynecology: a review of the literature. J Minim Invasive Gynecol 2019;26(2):327–43.

43. Meyer LA, Lasala J, Iniesta MD, et al. Effect of an enhanced recovery after surgery program on opioid use and patient-reported outcomes. Obstet Gynecol 2018;132(2):281–90.

44. Long JB, Bevil K, Giles DL. Preemptive analgesia in minimally invasive gynecologic surgery. J Minim Invasive Gynecol 2019;26(2):198–218.

45. Xiromeritis P, Kalogiannidis I, Papadopoulos E, et al. Improved recovery using multimodal perioperative analgesia in minimally invasive myomectomy: a randomised study. Aust N Z J Obstet Gynaecol 2011;51(4):301–6.

46. Gan TJ, Belani KG, Bergese S, et al. Fourth consensus guidelines for the management of postoperative nausea and vomiting. Anesth Analg 2020;131(2): 411–48.

47. Murphy GS, Szokol JW, Greenberg SB, et al. Preoperative dexamethasone enhances quality of recovery after laparoscopic cholecystectomy: effect on in-hospital and postdischarge recovery outcomes. Anesthesiology 2011;114(4): 882–90.

48. Committee Opinion No 701. Choosing the route of hysterectomy for benign disease. Obstet Gynecol 2017;129(6):e155–9.

49. Wechter ME, Mohd J, Magrina JF, et al. Complications in robotic-assisted gynecologic surgery according to case type: a 6-year retrospective cohort study using Clavien-Dindo classification. J Minim Invasive Gynecol 2014;21(5):844–50.

50. Penner KR, Fleming ND, Barlavi L, et al. Same-day discharge is feasible and safe in patients undergoing minimally invasive staging for gynecologic malignancies. Am J Obstet Gynecol 2015;212(2):186 e181–188.

51. Myriokefalitaki E, Smith M, Ahmed AS. Implementation of enhanced recovery after surgery (ERAS) in gynaecological oncology. Arch Gynecol Obstet 2016; 294(1):137–43.

52. Madani A, Fiore JF Jr, Wang Y, et al. An enhanced recovery pathway reduces duration of stay and complications after open pulmonary lobectomy. Surgery 2015;158(4):899–908, discussion 908-810.

53. Varadhan KK, Neal KR, Dejong CH, et al. The enhanced recovery after surgery (ERAS) pathway for patients undergoing major elective open colorectal surgery: a meta-analysis of randomized controlled trials. Clin Nutr 2010;29(4):434–40.

54. Song W, Wang K, Zhang RJ, et al. The enhanced recovery after surgery (ERAS) program in liver surgery: a meta-analysis of randomized controlled trials. Springerplus 2016;5:207.

55. Stowers MD, Manuopangai L, Hill AG, et al. Enhanced recovery after surgery in elective hip and knee arthroplasty reduces length of hospital stay. ANZ J Surg 2016;86(6):475–9.

56. Relph S, Bell A, Sivashanmugarajan V, et al. Cost effectiveness of enhanced recovery after surgery programme for vaginal hysterectomy: a comparison of pre

and post-implementation expenditures. Int J Health Plann Manage 2014;29(4): 399–406.

57. de Lapasse C, Rabischong B, Bolandard F, et al. Total laparoscopic hysterectomy and early discharge: satisfaction and feasibility study. J Minim Invasive Gynecol 2008;15(1):20–5.

58. Lassen PD, Moeller-Larsen H, Nulley PD. Same-day discharge after laparoscopic hysterectomy. Acta Obstet Gynecol Scand 2012;91(11):1339–41.

59. Rhou YJ, Pather S, Loadsman JA, et al. Direct hospital costs of total laparoscopic hysterectomy compared with fast-track open hysterectomy at a tertiary hospital: a retrospective case-controlled study. Aust N Z J Obstet Gynaecol 2015;55(6): 584–7.

# *Moving?*

## Make sure your subscription moves with you!

To notify us of your new address, find your **Clinics Account Number** (located on your mailing label above your name), and contact customer service at:

**Email: journalscustomerservice-usa@elsevier.com**

**800-654-2452** (subscribers in the U.S. & Canada)
**314-447-8871** (subscribers outside of the U.S. & Canada)

**Fax number: 314-447-8029**

**Elsevier Health Sciences Division**
**Subscription Customer Service**
**3251 Riverport Lane**
**Maryland Heights, MO 63043**

*To ensure uninterrupted delivery of your subscription, please notify us at least 4 weeks in advance of move.

9780323987455